# Psychoeducation Manual for Bipolar Disorder

Although the mainstay of bipolar therapy is drug treatment, psychoeducation is a technique that has proven to be very effective as an add-on to medication, helping to reduce the number of all types of bipolar recurrences and hospitalization. The object is to improve patients' understanding of the disorder and therefore their adherence to pharmacotherapy. Based on the highly successful, evidence-based Barcelona Program, this book is a pragmatic, therapist's guide for how to implement psychoeducation for bipolar patients. It gives practical guidance for how to conduct a psychoeducation group, using sessions and cases drawn from the Barcelona Psychoeducation Program. Moreover, it provides the reader with a great amount of practical tips and tricks, and specific techniques to maximize the benefits of bipolar psychoeducation.

The authors formed the first group to show the efficacy of psychoeducation as a maintenance treatment and have a long history of performing bipolar psychoeducation.

**Francesc Colom** is a Senior Researcher at the Bipolar Disorders Program, IDIBAPS, Hospital Clinic, Barcelona, and an Honorary Senior Lecturer at the Institute of Psychiatry, London.

**Eduard Vieta** is the Director of the Bipolar Disorders Program, IDIBAPS, Hospital Clinic, Barcelona, and a Professor of Psychiatry at the University of Barcelona.

GW00771773

# Psychoeducation Manual for Bipolar Disorder

**Francesc Colom**
Bipolar Disorder Program, IDIBAPS
Stanley Medical Research Center, Hospital Clinic, Barcelona

**Eduard Vieta**
Director, Bipolar Disorder Program, IDIBAPS
Stanley Medical Research Center, Hospital Clinic, Barcelona

**With a foreword by**

Jan Scott
Professor of Psychological Treatments Research
Institute of Psychiatry, London

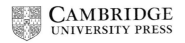

CAMBRIDGE
UNIVERSITY PRESS

CAMBRIDGE UNIVERSITY PRESS
Cambridge, New York, Melbourne, Madrid, Cape Town, Singapore, São Paulo

Cambridge University Press
The Edinburgh Building, Cambridge CB2 2RU, UK
Published in the United States of America by Cambridge University Press, New York

www.cambridge.org
Information on this title: www.cambridge.org/9780521683685

© Cambridge University Press 2006

This publication is in copyright. Subject to statutory exception
and to the provisions of relevant collective licensing agreements,
no reproduction of any part may take place without
the written permission of Cambridge University Press.

First published 2006
Typeset by Charon Tec Ltd (A Macmillan Company), Chennai, India
www.charontec.com

Printed in the United Kingdom at the University Press, Cambridge

*A catalogue record for this publication is available from the British Library*

*Library of Congress Cataloguing in Publication data*

ISBN-13 978-0-521-68368-5 paperback
ISBN-10 0-521-68368-8 paperback

Cambridge University Press has no responsibility for the persistence or accuracy of URLs for external or third-party Internet websites referred to in this publication, and does not guarantee that any content on such websites is, or will remain, accurate or appropriate.

Every effort has been made in preparing this publication to provide accurate and up-to-date information which is in accord with accepted standards and practice at the time of publication. Although case histories are drawn from actual cases, every effort has been made to disguise the identities of the individuals involved. Nevertheless, the authors, editors and publishers can make no warranties that the information contained herein is totally free from error, not least because clinical standards are constantly changing through research and regulation. The authors, editors and publishers therefore disclaim all liability for direct or consequential damages resulting from the use of material contained in this publication. Readers are strongly advised to pay careful attention to information provided by the manufacturer of any drugs or equipment that they plan to use.

**For Rosario and Gloria**

# Contents

# Foreword

More than perhaps for virtually any other mental illness, there is a need for a comprehensive and integrated approach to the management of bipolar disorders. The limited view that treatment of bipolar disorders consists only of finding the "right" pharmacotherapy has largely been dispelled. The availability of an array of medications proven to be beneficial in research trials has not changed the course of bipolar disorders as we encounter them in contemporary practice. Evidence suggests that this efficacy–effectiveness gap is a product, on the one hand, of the difficulty in getting bipolar patients to adhere to their medication treatment as prescribed and, on the other, a consequence of the greater prevalence of adverse psychological and social factors influencing the course of bipolar disorder in the heterogeneous populations treated in non-research clinical settings.

There is an increasing acceptance of the importance of the stress-vulnerability hypothesis as a model for understanding individual risk of relapse or poor prognosis in bipolar disorders. It is also accepted that patients' attitudes and beliefs about their disorder and its treatment influence how or whether they adjust to their predicament, and that this adjustment or lack of it will ultimately affect their outcome. Furthermore, helping the individual to recognize and change potentially harmful behaviors (such as drug or alcohol use), or encouraging the adoption of more stable and regular patterns of social activity (which may in turn stabilize circadian rhythms) are hypothesized as additional ways of reducing the risk of relapse. All of these research findings clearly indicated a role for an intervention that targets the psychosocial stressors that adversely affect outcome, and that help patients make informed choices about how to act or cope when faced with a long-term mental health problem. However, the dilemma confronting researchers in the field was what type of psychological intervention would meet all these requirements and would offer a complementary as opposed to a competing model of treatment. It is important that potential gains from a psychological therapy were not undermined because they reduced the patient's acceptance of the crucial role of mood stabilizers and other medications.

In the last decade, four main models of psychological interventions have evolved for bipolar disorders. Three (namely cognitive behavior therapy, interpersonal social rhythms therapy, and family-focused therapy) represent adaptations of evidence-based models previously applied successfully to the treatment of depression and/or schizophrenia. The fourth model was developed *de novo* by the Barcelona group. They adopted three key principles in devising their approach: (1) the intervention had to emphasize a psycho-bio-social model of bipolar disorders so that all treatment interventions, whether pharmacological or psychological, made sense (i.e. appeared rational) to the patient; (2) the program had to target the core psychosocial issues, and the interventions used must be evidence based (hence in common with the other approaches the core elements target adjustment, treatment adherence and reduction of substance misuse, regularization of social rhythms, and relapse prevention strategies); and (3) the program should give individuals specific and selected information about their disorder in a user-friendly format and also teach and allow practice of effective coping skills.

The unique aspects of the Barcelona approach are that it is based on the philosophy of psychoeducation, but uses an adult-learning model to achieve its goals, and it provides patients with a group approach which not only offers them peer support but also allows them to learn from each other. These elements are important. It is well known that information alone is a necessary but not sufficient method of changing behavior. Indeed many clinicians are cynical about psychoeducation because everyone claims to offer it to patients but few clinicians apply a systematic and comprehensive multifaceted model that helps individuals actually modify their actions or learn new coping or problem-solving skills. The psychoeducation program outlined in this manual clearly involves a carefully selected combination of information giving, guided self-learning and opportunities to develop and practice self-management skills under supervision. The sessions have a clear format that models to group members how to approach issues related to their mental health problems. The structure and containment provided by the mental health professionals ensures that the advantages of group learning and peer support are maximized. It is also clear that whilst the topics covered in this program are treated seriously, engagement and interaction with group members do not require the therapists to avoid humor, indeed there is a sub-text in this program that learning can also be an enjoyable process.

Those who know Francesc Colom and Eduard Vieta will be aware of the enormous international respect for their contributions to research on all aspects of bipolar disorders. This manual provides a detailed description of the approach used in their published studies of psychoeducation allowing replication of their program in research studies elsewhere and the translation of research into clinical practice. Clinicians practicing at other centers can now apply the group program developed in Barcelona. The information provided in the manual and the clarity of the session structure will also allow clinicians to institute any modifications required to meet the needs of local patient groups within the framework outlined, for example it is possible to accommodate variations in session content because of cultural differences or to integrate data on other treatments.

The needs of individuals with bipolar disorders are many and various. The program developed by the Catalan group is highly acceptable and readily understood by patients. It empowers them to engage in self-monitoring and self-management without ever undermining the importance of medication as a core component of the overall treatment package. Approaches that seamlessly integrate pharmacological and psychological approaches to bipolar disorders are few and far between, yet it is exactly these types of strategies that are urgently needed if we are to achieve better outcomes for our patients. The Barcelona group have made a critical contribution to clinical science and practice, and it is to their credit that they are also keen to share their program with colleagues who are also committed to improve the quality of life of individuals with bipolar disorders and their significant others.

**Jan Scott**
*Professor of Psychological Treatments Research,*
*Institute of Psychiatry, London, UK*

# Preface

In the days of the Roman Empire, after a military victory the Emperor would process in triumph before the excited and grateful crowds. The sun honored him from on high with the brightest of its rays, laurels wreathed his head, the centurions saluted him as a great leader, the plebeians venerated him, life smiled upon him, and the greatest glory was no more than a first step in his triumphal ascension to Deity. Behind him, part of his mighty retinue, walked the man. The man's job was to repeat systematically to the Emperor: "Remember you are not divine, remember you are human, remember you have to die."

This figure, real and fully documented by historians, perfectly illustrates the work of psychoeducation therapists: giving patients the information they need so they know where they are and can decide where to go.

When we started organizing psychoeducation groups for bipolar patients, very little information was available about this approach and there were no randomized trials with any degree of methodological rigor and no specific manual – so we had to draw on our knowledge of bipolar disorder and our own common sense. After some time had passed, a number of reviews and manuals started coming out, and we began to contact the pioneering researchers in this field. We were happy to see that almost all the teams, whether in the USA, Great Britain, The Netherlands, or Italy, were working toward the same goal, using similar techniques and looking at the same themes. In fact we came to similar conclusions. This was not surprising because the researchers had – and, we believe, still have – common sense and a certain clinical knowledge of bipolar disorders and, above all, because psychoeducation is an intervention whose need is obvious in the case of bipolar patients. But being obvious or commonsensical does not necessarily mean that it has to be efficacious. One of the functions of the scientific method is precisely to prove the obvious, and happily psychoeducation has abundantly demonstrated its efficacy in prevention of relapses in bipolar disorders – something we are proud to say because our group has played a significant role.

This book is a manual for teaching your patients to manage their disorder better, live with it, progress with it, take their medication more effectively, and understand why the medication needs to be taken. But above all, it is a teaching manual for a technique that will help your bipolar patients suffer fewer relapses.

This book will give you the tools you need to run a psychoeducation program which is not only absolutely essential from the standpoint of evidence-based medicine but is also a right of the patient – the right to know more about his disorder – and a vital backup for the medication.

We designed this book to be practical and easy to use. We begin with a general introduction on the clinical presentation of bipolar disorders and a brief review of psychological interventions tried to date; we then look at why the use of psychoeducation in bipolar disorder is important and what its action mechanisms are, then talk about the formal aspects of our intervention – duration, frequency, format, etc. After these theoretical and practical introductory topics, we go on to describe in each of the five units our intervention which consists of 21 sessions, with a specific chapter for each session. Each chapter in turn is appropriately broken down into five sections:

- *Goal of session*: The concrete goal of a given session is described.
- *Procedure*: The steps to be taken in each session are described in detail.
- *Useful tips*: This section will give the clinician useful tips to help run the session – all based on our direct experience in psychoeducation work.
- *Patient materials*: These are the updated materials distributed to patients at the end of the session so that the reader can use them in his or her clinical practice. We recommend that the psychologist or psychiatrist who is thinking about running a psychoeducation program will keep these kinds of materials constantly updated.
- *Assignments*: After the materials, we have included the assignments we give to the patients for the forthcoming week. Since the assignments are meant to be prepared for the next session in some way, each assignment refers to the content of the following week's session.

We believe this structure will make it easier to use the book and apply our program.

Now back to the man who talked to the Emperor. What must still be said is that his future in those days would involve not only the separation between the body and the mind – a common mistake in the psychology of yesteryear – but rather between the body and the head, an intervention that usually caused the death of the individual. We hope our future will be a brighter one, without forgetting that we shall one day die.

**Francesc Colom**
**Eduard Vieta**

# Part 1

# Clinical, diagnostic, and therapeutic aspects of bipolar disorders

# Introduction

Bipolar disorders, classically known as "manic–depressive psychosis," is a serious, chronic, and relapsing mental disorder. Despite the growing efficacy of available pharmacological tools, bipolar-affective disorders have continued to be a significant source of morbidity and mortality, doing serious harm to the quality of life of sufferers. They are the sixth cause of disability worldwide (López and Murray, 1998) and, serious and chronic as they are, represent a heavy financial and social burden – both direct (hospitalizations and consumption of medical resources) and indirect (constant days missed from work and loss of productivity) (Wyatt and Henter, 1995; Goetzel et al., 2003).

The incidence of bipolar disorders amounts to approximately 4% of the adult population (Hirschfeld et al., 2003), but may reach 6.5% of the population at large if minor and atypical forms are included (Angst, 1995). The consequences of the disorder and its subsequent relapses for the individual and for family members, combined with the high risk of mortality by suicide (Vieta et al., 1992, 1997a, b, c; Tsai et al., 2002) suggest that a multiple therapeutic effort must be made, going beyond while at the same time supportive of drug therapy.

# Bipolar disorders through history

The first references to mania and melancholia go back to Araeteus of Capadocia in the second century BC. For centuries, the term "mania" was used to refer to agitation syndromes, whatever their origin. The first attempts to find a solid biological substrate for mania arose with the liberalization of cadaver dissection and the advent of the anatomical–clinical methods. However, it was not until the nineteenth century that the concepts of mania and depression were linked conceptually and clinically through the first detailed descriptions of the *folie circulaire* by Falret and the *folie à double forme* by Baillarger – both the conditions characterized by states of excitation, sadness, and lucid intervals of variable duration. The introduction of recurrence and the cyclicity to descriptions of the disorder is one of the breakthrough moments in the history of psychiatry, and even discussion of the authorship of the concept makes quite an interesting story (Pichot, 1995). Falret and Baillarger simultaneously, in 1854, described the cyclicity of the disorder. These two doctors worked in the same city (Paris), were of similar age, and were the disciples of a single master, Esquirol, who had actually taught almost all French psychiatrists of the era. They kept up a brisk polemic about who was first to define the concept, each claiming to have described it first, albeit as part of lectures given to young medical students (in the case of Falret) or in a clinical session at the Academy of Medicine (Baillarger). What is certain is that this polemic took over their lives and poisoned their personal relationship. The gulf could not be bridged even when the two met face to face at a conference on February 14, 1854. As stubborn as they were brilliant, each persisted in the conviction that he was first, and the other was the upstart. The story had a happy, somewhat bitter–sweet, ending when Falret's son, also a psychiatrist and the successor of Baillarger, settled the dispute after the deaths of the two savants. With the wisdom of a Solomon but somewhat gratuitously, he attributed the genesis of the idea to both, and in a fine gesture started a fund-raising campaign to erect a monument to Baillarger. On July 7, 1894, the French, masters of the subtle art of diplomacy, concluded what they rather high-mindedly called "a battle between giants" in a ceremony presided over by the busts of the two geniuses, who observed the evolution of mental disorders from the gardens of the most prestigious psychiatrist in Paris. The contest ended in a draw, and was a major step forward for psychiatry.

Much earlier, in the eighteenth century, although far more anecdotally, the Spanish doctor Piquer Arrufat described the disease of King Ferdinand VI as a mania–melancholia. Arrufat's writings, fortunately revived in a fine new edition prepared by Vieta and Barcia (2000), are seasoned with moments of great clinical wisdom and inspiration (almost surprising for his time), and with curiosities, particularly with regard to the treatments essayed.

But the one who truly defined the outlines of the disorder by introducing the longitudinal study as an essential diagnostic tool was Emil Kraepelin whose work *Manic–Depressive Insanity and Paranoia* was a watershed in setting out the nosological aspects of bipolar disorders. He drew the boundaries of manic–depressive psychosis with schizophrenia, described the episodic course of the disorder, formulated its inheritability, and characterized its main clinical forms. Kraepelin's work was followed and extensively developed by psychiatrists in Europe, although less so in North America which was influenced more by the ideas of Adolf Meyer and the psychoanalysts who fled Europe with the advent of Nazism.

Almost as important as the work of Kraepelin were the studies by Leonhard, who postulated a separation between bipolar and unipolar forms of affective disorders from clinical, evolutional, and familial differences. This division was independently validated by Angst and Perris in 1966. Their studies, together with those of the North American group led by George Winokur, became the scientific and clinical basis for the early classifications of affective disorders based on the use of standardized criteria.

In parallel to the evolution in nosological concepts, the history of bipolar disorders is marked by the discovery of lithium salts. Lithium was tested on human beings for the first time in 1949 when the Australian scientist, John Cade, described its "tranquilizing" properties. Next, Scandinavian psychiatrists, especially the Mogens Schou group, conducted the first clinical trials and demonstrated its antimanic activity. Due to its molecular simplicity and therapeutic specificity, lithium continues to be a fascinating drug and its prophylactic effect has not been surpassed even today.

# Diagnosis and classification

The diagnosis of bipolar disorders and its episodes is based on purely clinical criteria which are hence subject to controversy and interpretation. Nonetheless, bipolar disorders (especially type I) has in its favor a validity of construct and long-term stability that are greater than those of other mental disorders. Unlike anxiety, depression, or psychosis, mania is one of the most specific concepts in psychiatric nosology. The *Diagnostic and Statistical Manual for Mental Disorders 4th edition* (DSM-IV) diagnostic criteria for schizophrenia require exclusion of a manic picture, but the reverse is not the case. Even so, maniform symptoms are observed in other pathologies.

In its time, DSM-IV had some novel features over the 3rd revised edition, DSM-III-R: incorporation of type II bipolar disorders as a category of its own, including cases previously classified as unspecified bipolar disorders; inclusion in the affective disorder section of substance-induced mood disorders or organic illness; and incorporation of a series of specifications with prognostic value. Some of these specifications are:

- "with catatonic characteristics," a specification added because many catatonic presentations are associated with mood disorders rather than with schizophrenia;
- "with atypical characteristics," meaning a depressive phase characterized by mood reactivity, reverse vegetative symptoms and hypersensitivity to rejection, and were probably incorporated with a view to their therapeutic implications; and
- "postpartum-initiated," a specification indicating a better prognosis but with particular vulnerability to recurring with each childbirth.

Longitudinal-course specifications were also incorporated to give information on the degree of interepisodic recovery. Rapid cycling was also recognized, in view of its poorer prognosis, poor response to lithium, and risks of anti-depressant treatment in these patients. The seasonality and melancholic symptom criteria were slightly modified. Other changes had to do with the duration of the mania and hypomania symptoms, and the classification of pharmacogenic manias and hypomanias as substance-induced syndromes, although this is without doubt one aspect that needs to improve: in view of the non-specificity of some symptoms, future psychiatric taxonomists will have to include loser temporal criteria or withdraw these temporal criteria in order not to under-diagnose and hence leave untreated many of those affected by the less classical forms of disorder entities. In this sense, the future criteria for hypomania should look at the possibility of including episodes lasting less than 4 days – a time limit that certainly has no empirical support. A number of studies support this argument and argue for broadening the bipolar spectrum (Akiskal et al., 2000; Benazzi, 2001). On the other hand, more attention needs to be paid to the role of ethnocultural variables in the presentation of manic symptomatology, which often mask it and make diag-nosis difficult, especially if we are talking about hypomania (Kirmayer and Groleau, 2001). All these may lead us to consider hypomania as a far more frequent syndrome than what has been established thus far, with a prevalence of up to 6.5% (Angst, 1998), and to bear in mind the possibility of it present-ing in a mild form in which cognition plays a key role (Colom et al., 2002).

The WHO classification, the International Classification of Disease, 10th edition (ICD-10), is fairly similar but does not include cyclothymia in the definition of bipolar disorders; also, cases of unipolar mania and type II bipolar disorders are classified in a residual category ("other bipolar disor-ders"). It is also certain, however, that some preliminary criteria were intro-duced for incorporating type II bipolar disorders, likely to be in a specific category in the 11th edition of the ICD.

## Cross-sectional diagnosis

### Manic phase

As we know, the basic symptomatology of the manic phase of bipolar disor-ders is defined from a limited period of time in which there is a mood change featuring not only euphoria but also expansiveness and irritability, with accompanying symptoms including excessive self-esteem or grandiosity (which can be delusional), reduced sleep, logorrhea, racing thoughts, distractibility, increased involvement in pleasurable or high-risk activities while disdaining them, and psychomotor anxiety or agitation. In distinguishing it from hypomania, it is felt that in mania the change must be serious enough to bring about a sharp deterioration in sufferers' social/job activity, or to require them to be hospitalized so that they are protected from hurting themselves or others. Other associated symptoms may be emotional lability, anxiety, and dysphoria. When there are hallucinations or delusional ideas, the content is usually, but not always, related to mood. In fact, there is mounting evidence that symptoms traditionally considered exclusive to schizophrenia are present in bipolar patients during a severe manic episode (McElroy et al., 1996). Among these symptoms, which can be even more frequent than the so-called "mood-congruent" symptoms (Tohen et al., 1992) are Kurt Schneider's first-rank symptoms. In ICD-10, these patients are classified as schizoaffective. This is one of the most fundamental sources of diagnostic confusion between schizophrenia and manic–depressive psychosis – a confusion that may affect about one-fourth of bipolar patients (Vieta et al., 1994).

## Hypomanic phase

The characteristic picture of hypomanic episodes consists of a predominantly elevated, expansive, or irritable mood, and actual manic symptoms for a given period of time, but not to a degree such that there is a marked deterioration in social or job performance, or such as to require hospitalization. In general, all the symptoms tend to be milder than in mania, and there is no psychotic symptomatology. Hypomania is a difficult syndrome to detect, especially with hindsight, and the difficulties in its diagnosis are the main source of errors in identifying type II bipolar disorder, which is confused with unipolar disorder and personality disorders. The borderline between hypomania and nonpathological elevated emotions is difficult to pin down, especially in highly educated individuals. Certain patterns of socially positive behavior (extreme sociability, good organizational skills, unstoppable decision-making and drive) are combined with the pathological expression of altered mood. The problem with such apparently virtuous hypomania is that the patient says she or he is making up for lost time, which is the strongest predictor of the next depressive episode.

From a more psychological standpoint, the cognitive–behavioral model has proven useful thus far in explaining cognitive function in depression

(Beck, 1976) and, more recently, the implications of cognitive features such as self-esteem (Winters and Neale, 1985), attributional style, coping skills (Lam and Wong, 1997), and the decision-making process (Murphy et al., 2001) in bipolar disorders. The cognitive model fits perfectly into the medical model of the disorder, without discussing it and complementing it, partly because its great research tradition makes it easily testable empirically. Here it is very interesting to single out studies that find cognitive vulnerability in bipolar patients that is qualitatively and quantitatively similar to that of unipolar depressive patients (Scott et al., 2000b).

The cognitive model of mania (Colom et al., 2002) fully assumes that it is organically based and, taking a somewhat more than descriptive approach, points to the existence of distorted thinking, as occurs with depression. Mania, however, is characterized by a "positive" cognitive triad: over-optimistic view of oneself, the world, and the future. Manic-automatic thoughts are positive cognitions and interpretations that do not square with reality. As with depression, these are rigid, inflexible, and unrealistic thoughts (Colom et al., 2002). Beyond these suppositions, we feel that cognitions play a key role in hypomania, both as a triggering or aggravating factor and as a therapeutic tool designed to improve three aspects in particular: (a) organization of behavior, that is reduction of stimuli, postponing decisions, increasing the sleep pattern; (b) analysis of cognitions; and (c) improvement in therapeutic adherence, traditionally poor in bipolar patients. The superiority of this approach to dynamic and psychogenic models is due to the fact that it is less reductionist to a psychological model, so that it can be adjusted and combined with the medical/biological approach. At the present time, there is definite evidence that certain behavioral interventions can bring about biological changes; for example, it has been shown that sleep deprivation can bring on hypomania (Wehr et al., 1982). This phenomenon has been described, albeit anecdotally, for cognitive therapy (Kingdon et al., 1986).

The presence of cognitive changes during hypomania and depression phases is indubitable, and forms part of its diagnostic criteria. However, just as nihilistic, fatalistic thinking and underevaluation of one's own capabilities should be understood not as a causal factor of depression but as a symptom of depression, the positive thinking characteristic of hypomania must also be considered a symptom, not a cause. The presence of changes in the method of processing information during a hypomanic episode has an etiologic value *per se*, so that it must be recognized as playing an important role when "nourishing" the severity of the symptoms, as cognitive changes generally involve behavioral changes and the latter do aggravate an episode, beginning an actual hypomanic spiral that feeds on itself. This is why detection of cognitive changes has a great therapeutic value favoring early intervention in hypomanic phases when the spiral is less powerful. The states of emotional exaltation triggered by substances or physical diseases would be a good model, or at any rate the least bad model, for interpreting the cognitive changes that occur during a hypomanic episode (Vieta and Cirera, 1997). The effects of stimulants, for example, may mimic some of the phenomena observable in hypomanic patients, although the short duration of the elating effect prevents the cognitive changes from settling in and progressing.

To describe such cognitive changes in isolation is no easy task, as they appear to be an interwoven whole and do not usually exist independently. Some of them would be quantitative (i.e. consist of accentuation of a feature that was also present in asymptomatic periods) and others would be qualitative (i.e. would correspond to "new" modes of thinking for the patient). Thus, it is easier to describe a cognitive style qualitatively characteristic of the hypomanic phases, which we decided to call "anastrophic thinking" by contrast to the catastrophic thinking of depressive phases. This particular way of processing information would basically include overevaluation of the ego, a positive interpretation of reality, and unwarranted, disproportionate, and uncritical optimism.

The intrusive behaviors of hypomanic periods are strongly connected to the above-mentioned cognitive changes and in their turn contribute to worsening the patient's condition. Just as Beck (1979) defines some "depressogenic" suppositions which by themselves and by modifying the subject's behavior aggravate depressive symptoms, we would venture to propose, based on the Beck model itself, the existence of an "elatogenic" hypothesis (from the Greek *elata*, which Kahlbaum connects to thymic exaltation as distinct from *melana*, the root of the term "melancholia"). The existence of these concepts would be linked to the presence of an exalted mood that would be part of a psychobiological process whose presence would give rise to a series of anastrophic and anastrogenic cognitions.

Trying to establish a causal order between emotional, cognitive, and behavioral states beyond the contingency itself is virtually impossible without falling back somewhat on theoretical speculation. What is certain is that there appears to exist a feedback process between emotion and cognition, a process that affects behavior which eventually closes the cycle, modifying certain biological aspects through, for example, sleep deprivation. This cycle starts up again with the severity of the syndrome increasing each time with a snowball effect, increasing in size and speed to a veritable avalanche. A clear example of this phenomenon is the absence of fatigue in the manic patient; the greater the number of stimuli and activity, the more she or he becomes involved in them and the less time she or he spends asleep, this creating a vicious cycle with a crescendo effect on the symptomatology.

## Depressive phase

The depressive phase of bipolar disorders has some features that distinguish it from unipolar endogenous depression on the one hand and reactive or situational depression on the other hand. The depressive phase of manic–depressive disorder is often accompanied by apathy predominating over sadness, psychomotor inhibition over anxiety, and hypersomnia over insomnia. Another difference described in the literature on bipolar and unipolar depressions is that, in the former, there is less anorexia and weight loss while emotional lability and the probability of developing psychotic symptoms in severe cases are greater. Epidemiologically, the age at which the disorder begins, in bipolar depression sufferers is younger and the incidence of postpartum episodes is greater. Other differences characteristic of bipolar forms are a family history of mania and completed suicide, and good response to lithium (Dunner, 1980). In young patients, the presence of catatonic stupor is frequent, and in the elderly, pseudodementia is likewise frequent.

## Mixed phase

Mixed states are characterized by the simultaneous appearance of manic and depressive symptoms in different combinations, depending on mood swings, and cognitive and behavioral changes. The most common form, called depressive mania, is a picture characterized by hyperactivity and psychomotor anxiety, global insomnia, tachypsychia, and logorrhea, combined with depressive thinking, weeping and emotional lability, and often-delusional guilt feelings, all of which can be in various combinations. With the present criteria of DSM-IV, the appearance of a mixed state necessarily carries the diagnosis of type I bipolar disorders, as it is at least as severe as mania. Doubt remains, however, as to whether attenuated forms of mixed episodes or mixed hypomanias are possible.

Mixed states are difficult to diagnose and treat, and are usually associated with a high risk of suicide.

## Longitudinal diagnosis: classification

### Type I bipolar disorders

Type I bipolar disorders correspond to the classical pattern of the disorder, and its basic distinguishing feature is the presence of mania. The most frequent pattern is mania followed by major depression. The psychotic symptoms can appear both in the manic phase and in the depressive phase, but may also be absent. The main difficulties in differential diagnosis occur with schizophrenia, probably through over-evaluation of florid psychotic symptoms such as those considered "first rank" by Kurt Schneider, and because the proper attention has not been paid to the prior course of the disorder.

### Type II bipolar disorders

Type II bipolar disorders consist of a combination of major depressive episodes with spontaneous hypomanias. The scientific community is divided between those who feel that depressed patients with hypomania linked to antidepressant treatment should be classified as type II bipolar and those who prefer to classify then as unipolar with substance-induced hypomanic episodes, an option corresponding to the DSM-IV classification. Type II bipolar disorders are a valid category, distinct from type I bipolar disorders and unipolar disorder in genetic, biological, clinical, outcome-related, and pharmacological aspects (Menchón et al., 1993). The pioneering work of Ayuso and Ramos (1982) noted the fact, as was borne out by later studies, that although type II is associated with greater clinical benignancy, it often proves to be less benign as it evolves, in the sense of a larger number of episodes. Although this is a fairly stable category, between 5% and 15% of those affected have at least one manic episode and thus become type I bipolar patients (Coryell et al., 1995). Many type II bipolar patients are diagnosed and treated as if they were unipolar patients, because the patient only goes to the doctor when she or he is depressed. All depressed patients should be asked, if possible with family input, about any history of hypomania. Type II bipolar disorders could be one of the categories with greater comorbidity and higher risk of suicide.

## Cyclothymia

Cyclothymia is considered a minor variant of bipolar disorders and often evolves into type II or, more often, type I. According to Akiskal, echoing Kraepelin, cyclothymia constitutes the temperamental substrate of bipolar disorders. It is characterized by a chronic course and a high frequency of episodes, to the point that DSM-IV holds the absence of episodes for only 2 months to be an exclusion criterion. The episodes are mild in intensity but extremely frequent, and the behavioral changes that accompany them involve psychosocial complications. Many cyclothymic patients are diagnosed with borderline personality disorders. In some cases there is comorbidity with adult attention-deficit hyperactivity disorders. These patients are characteristically resistant to antidepressant treatments, especially with tricyclics, but also with monoamine oxidase (MAO) inhibitors, and respond better to mood stabilizers.

## Other bipolar disorders

Some authors have proposed new categorical subtypes such as type III bipolar disorders (Akiskal et al., 2000) for patients with family histories of bipolar disorders who had depression and hypomania only during the antidepressant treatment. The same author defends the existence of patients with hyperthymic temperaments who experience depression episodes having psychobiological features closer to the bipolar spectrum than the unipolar, and anxious depressions that could be considered mixed states. At the other extreme, schizoaffective disorders and cycloid psychoses could be part of the spectrum, although the former have a recognized place in the two existing taxonomies.

# Psychological interventions in bipolar disorders

The possible role of psychological interventions in the treatment of bipolar disorders has followed a course comparable with that of type I bipolar disorders itself, with psychotic symptoms in both the phases. After an initial phase of grandiose psychoanalytic euphoria, in which it was assumed that psychotherapy would play a fundamental role in the treatment of bipolar disorders and that words – or in some cases the absence of words – would "cure" this disorder, neurobiological and pharmacological findings appeared to usher in a serious melancholic phase for psychotherapy in the mid-1970s and 1980s; this age was open not only to pesimism, but to speculation, and just a few open studies with small samples were published. Optimism for psychotherapy in bipolar disorders returned in the 1990s due to two factors:

1   the availability of new drugs effective in treating the disorder, spurring renewed interest in clinical research and treatment;
2   the evidence that certain psychological interventions had proven highly effective in conjunction with drugs for other disorders, such as schizophrenia.

As a result, several teams worldwide refocused on applying psychotherapy to bipolar disorders. Reviews and manuals began to come out in the mid-1990s, and rigorous randomized clinical studies on the usefulness of various techniques began to appear in 1999.

The psychological interventions proposed for bipolar disorders in the course of history are highly diverse, but the majority of them were published without adequate methodological support, without control groups or blinded reviews of results, and based only on anecdotal descriptions that are difficult to extrapolate (Swartz and Frank, 2001). Also, the absence of independent analyses for each clinical or progressive subtype of the disorder makes the results difficult to interpret.

## Psychoanalysis

Throughout history, the relationship between psychoanalysis and the bipolar patient has not been an especially smooth one – at least, this is what its early psychoanalytic writings seem to show: Abraham (1911) defined bipolar patients as "impatient, envious, exploitive …" and later, in 1949, Fromm-Reichmann referred to them as "incredibly skilled" at detecting vulnerabilities on the part of the therapist. Other authors considered that bipolar patients tended to bring about a "strong countertransference" in the analyst (Rosenfeld, 1963), which is readily understandable if we think about the illusion of control over symptoms that psychoanalysis developed with regard to bipolar disorders, and if we think about the causal explanations of mania and the poor fit of all the above with reality, evidenced by the fact that any patient treated with psychoanalysis alone will not only experience an improvement but, if adequate pharmacological treatment is not received, will probably suffer a relapse in the course of the disorder. In this case –in most cases, in fact – "frustration" would be a good synonym for "countertransference."

## Group therapy

It has always been considered that bipolar patients were unsuitable members of therapy groups; in fact they have been defined as "one of the worst calamities that could befall group therapy" (Yalom, 1995). Happily, thanks to initiatives such as the National Depressive and Manic–Depressive Association of the USA, in the past 15 years there has been an increasing trend to form groups of bipolar patients as a method of improving drug adherence, educating patients about the disorder, destigmatization, and solving the problems involved in bipolar disorders; these groups are based on a psychoeducation approach.

The study by Shakir et al. (1979), using group therapy as a supplement to lithium treatment, deserves special mention. Psychological treatment combined attention to therapeutic adherence with interpersonal therapy centered on here and now. After 2 years of follow-up, the outcomes of patients receiving group therapy improved to a great degree. A subsequent follow-up (Volkmar et al., 1981) showed a clear reduction in the hospitalization rates of patients treated with group therapy plus lithium. There was also increased adherence with lithium treatment, attributed to the interaction between the direct group effect and closer monitoring.

As time passed, a trend consolidated toward more directive group therapy models. Thus, Kripke and Robinson (1985), for example, based their group therapy on problem-solving strategies and checked plasma lithium levels to ensure drug adherence. The relapse rate and social adjustment improved.

In 1986, Foelker et al. designed the first psychotherapeutic program for elderly bipolar patients from an integration of traditional therapeutic approaches and psychoeducation, monitoring of lithium levels, and case management. Especially, interesting is the inclusion in the group therapy of the effects of the disorder on social adjustment and the interpersonal aspects of dealing with it (Wulsin et al., 1988). Other authors (Pollack, 1995) suggest that group therapy should begin during hospitalization, even during the acute phase. The group also offers a safe, controlled setting that can cushion shocks during stressful periods (Spitz, 1988). Likewise, group therapy allows negation mechanisms to be effectively challenged (Graves, 1993). Although we do not yet have scientific evidence on the point, we believe that the combination of group therapy and the psychoeducation approach is the best strategy if patients are to adequately manage their disorder and its consequences, improve their social and interpersonal adjustment, and obtain the maximum benefit from each intervention. To achieve these results, one of the basic objectives of group therapy should be adherence with drug prescriptions (Paykel, 1995). It has been demonstrated that the Life-Goals Program for bipolar patients of Bauer and McBride (1996), which is structured group psychotherapy expressly designed for manic–depressive disorder, is able to decrease the utilization of emergency services and their associated costs (Bauer, 1997). This program has two phases: (i) one of which is basically psychoeducative and (ii) the other focuses on working out realistic steps to achieve goals that are significant for the subject. Group intervention has also been tested from a cognitive perspective (Patelis-Siotis et al., 2001), although to date the results have not been conclusive.

## Interpersonal therapy

The results of interpersonal therapy, an approach developed by Gerald Klerman and his team (Klerman et al., 1984) can be evaluated as simply and reliably as the results of drug treatment. It is a limited-time type of therapy centering on psychosocial and interpersonal problems and bringing in psychoanalytic concepts (in fact it was originally an adaptation of Sullivan's dynamic interpersonal therapy) as well as cognitive and behavioral concepts. It does not claim to rebuild the personality, at least during the symptomatic stage, but emphasizes reaffirmation, clarification of emotional states, improvement in interpersonal communications, objectivization of perceptions, and adequate performance in interpersonal situations (Klerman, 1988). Originally designed to treat depression, basically to identify the triggers of this disorder, its application has broadened to other disorders. Subsequently, the Pittsburgh group (Frank et al., 1990) developed interpersonal maintenance therapy, then renamed interpersonal social rhythm therapy, in order to improve prevention of relapses in recovered patients. Its effectiveness in treating depression has already been demonstrated (Frank et al., 1991) but this is not the case for bipolar disorders. The Pittsburgh group is currently working on this issue through introduction of various specific changes (Ehlers et al., 1988; Frank et al., 1994). The classical study by Frank et al. (1990) was the first to demonstrate that psychological intervention was more effective than placebo in treating patients with recurrent unipolar depression. However, the results of combining interpersonal psychotherapy and antidepressant drugs were no better than drug treatment alone (Kupfer et al., 1992).

The latest advances in interpersonal therapy applied to bipolar patients (Frank et al., 1994, 2000) tend to integrate the chrono-biological and interpersonal approaches into a single model that could be useful both during and acute episodes and for prevention of relapses. This treatment is a combination of interpersonal and cognitive–behavioral techniques. The classical interpersonal techniques, for example evocation of affect and analysis of relationships and communication, are used to resolve grief reactions, and interpersonal discussions are used to improve interpersonal deficits and negotiate role changes. Behavioral techniques, for example log-keeping, goal-setting, gradual assignment of tasks, and cognitive restructuring, are used to regularize lifestyles and establish social rhythms. Emphasis on chrono-biological factors is due to the abundance of studies on the role these factors play in relapse, basically through sleep deprivation (Wehr et al., 1987).

On the other hand, it has been reported that social rhythm therapy – an intervention combining the basic principles of interpersonal psychotherapy and behavioral techniques to help patients regularize their daily routines, reduce interpersonal problems, and adhere to dosing regimens – is effective in treating some aspects of bipolar disorders (Frank et al., 2000).

## Cognitive–behavioral therapy

Interventions of the cognitive–behavioral type are without a shadow of a doubt those with the greatest tradition in the treatment of affective disorders, especially in unipolar depression, in which their efficacy has been demonstrated on repeated occasions. They are used in combination therapy or as monotherapy, and as prophylactic treatment (Fava et al., 1998; Jarrett et al., 2001) – although there are also studies with negative results (Perlis et al., 2002) – as treatment of acute phases (Keller et al., 2000; Ward et al., 2000) in various types of residual depression (Fava et al., 1996; Scott et al., 2000a), atypical depression (Jarrett et al., 1999), and recurrent depression (Blackburn and Moore, 1997) where monotherapy with cognitive treatment has even proved superior to drug treatment. This is to the degree that some authors suggest that the term "resistant depression" should not be used until cognitive therapy has been tried as therapeutic alternative (Fava et al., 1997).

These efficacy studies cannot be extrapolated to bipolar depression; for one thing it is subtly different from unipolar depression (Mitchel and Malhi, 2005). Some studies tell us that bipolar depression is usually more uninhibited than unipolar depression, with fatigue, hypersomnia, and apathy being the predominant symptoms. In fact, it appears that behavioral symptomatology is more evident than cognitive symptomatology. Experts in cognitive–behavioral therapy (CBT) have often been unaware of this factor and have tried to adapt the classical Beck model to bipolar depression (Leahy and Beck, 1988), without significant results. The idea behind cognitive therapy is that mood swings are caused in part by negative thinking patterns, and these patterns can be modified by behavioral activation and cognitive restructuring. The subtle problem of this classical framing of CBT in its adaptation to bipolar disorders is that it is not certain that cognitions actually guide affective changes, at least in the majority of patients. What is more, in some patients there is not even a cognitive change specific to bipolar depression beyond the person's own desperation after a period of instability; that is, the cognitive change, if there is one, is a consequence of depression rather than its cause. Let us not forget that many depressed bipolar patients do not have the cognitive distortions typical of unipolar depressions, but do have a feeling of affective vacuum or blank mood. In our opinion, to respond to the actual needs of the depressed bipolar patient, the psychotherapy of bipolar depression must emphasize the behavioral rather than the cognitive.

With respect to cognitive intervention in bipolar disorders, to date its feasibility in bipolar disorders has been successfully studied (Palmer and Williams, 1995; Patelis-Siotis et al., 2001) and its efficacy in prevention of all sorts of recurrences (Lam et al., 2003). Previously, cognitive intervention had shown efficacy in improved adherence with treatment (Cochran, 1984). However, the efficacy of this type of intervention in treatment of bipolar depression has not yet been conclusively tested, although there are high-quality, well-structured manuals (Lam et al., 1999). In one open study, Fava et al. (2001) showed the efficacy of CBT in prevention of episodes, although the results of this study should be interpreted with caution due to the small size of the sample ($N = 15$) and the nonexistence of a control group. The study of Dominic Lam (2003) using quite a large sample (103 patients) shows the efficacy of cognitive therapy in the prevention of depressive and manic episodes, in the shortening of depressive phases, and in the reduction of subdepressive symptomatology (Lam et al., 2003). In addition, this therapy could be useful for treating postepisodic dysphoria in which the patient often feels guilty about what she or he did during the manic phase and what she or he did not do during the depressive phase (Jacobs, 1982). However, the biggest CBT study performed until now offers contradictory results, as CBT may even worsen the outcome of bipolar disorder in those patients with a longer disorder evolution (Scott et al., 2006). The cognitive–behavioral approach in a group also showed some efficacy in cases of dual pathology, for example in substance-abuse/dependency disorders comorbid with bipolar disorder; in a 6-month study on treatment with CBT in conjunction with drug treatment, after 3 months follow-up, an improvement in substance-taking disorders was observed in patients with this type of comorbidity and also a reduction in the number of manic relapses, but not of depressive relapses (Weiss et al., 2000).

The Beck group (Leahy and Beck, 1988) defined the use of classical cognitive techniques (e.g. analysis of cognitive errors in information processing or analysis of the behavioral consequences of specific actions) to treat depression and hypomania. The work of Basco and Rush (1996) incorporates elements of CBT and psychoeducation to try to increase the degree of adherence with the lithium prescription, as well as to help patients recognize dysfunctional information-processing patterns and prevent relapses – although this proposal has not been properly tested. Some of these authors use classical cognitive–behavioral techniques, such as writing down symptoms and problem-solving and confrontation strategies; their therapeutic implementation has a great deal of overlap with psychoeducation and can even be considered a subtype of behaviorally oriented psychoeducation.

## Family intervention in bipolar patients

Bipolar disorders affect not only the patient but also those who lives with, who actually suffers the consequences of the disorder as well as taking over in the caregiver role. Dore and Romans (2001) pointed out the impact of living with bipolar patients on caregivers in areas such as job, finances, legal aspects, couple relationships, marital relationships, caring for children, social relationships, and leisure activities. A number of studies have found that the burdens borne by families of bipolar patients are heavy (Chakrabarti et al., 1992; Perlick et al., 1999). These findings take on even more significance with the results of the Perlick et al. (2001) study reporting that the caregiver's burden could predict the clinical outcome of patients with this disorder.

It is obvious from all the above that the patient's disorder and family functioning interact with each other. The degree of environmental stress in the course of bipolar disorders, the burden experienced by the family members living with the patient, and the demands by families for more information on the disorder and strategies for dealing with it are some of the reasons behind the introduction of psychoeducative interventions centered on the family of the bipolar patient (Reinares et al., 2002a). To date, a number of studies have suggested that family intervention together with drug treatment is an effective resource for improving the outcomes of bipolar patients. Family intervention of the psychoeducation type sets out to provide families with knowledge that helps them improve their understanding of the disorder, and make certain changes in their attitudes and behaviors to optimize strategies for dealing with the disorder (Reinares et al., 2002b).

Some studies have reported the effect of family intervention on reducing the number of relapses (Miklowitz and Goldstein, 1990; Miklowitz et al., 2000) or admissions (Davenport, 1977). The Miklowitz et al. (2000) study is remarkable for its methodological rigor: after an acute episode, a number of bipolar patients were randomly assigned to family intervention ($N = 31$) consisting of psychoeducation, training in communications skills, and training in problem-solving, or classical treatment with two educational sessions ($N = 70$). The results suggest that family intervention reduces the number of relapses and improves depression symptoms, although not mania symptoms. The most substantial changes were found in emotionally expressive families.

Subsequent studies from the same group (Miklowitz et al., 2003) indicate that family psychoeducation can also increase the interval to the next hospitalization and improve therapeutic adherence. Our own group also identified psychoeducation in families as a very useful tool for reducing the impact of the disorder on the family (Reinares et al., in press).

**Part 2**

# Concept and methodology of psychoeducation

# Psychological treatment and bipolar disorders: why psychoeducate?

The primary purpose of any treatment, whether psychological or pharmaco-logical, should always be the curing of a disorder, or at least an improving of the symptoms. Thus, we should be very critical of those treatments that offer only improvements of secondary aspects, like quality of life, or unspecific results, like the patient's subjective evaluation of the treatment in question. The latter is especially common for psychological treatments. Thus, it can be said that most psychological treatments might be useless because, perhaps due to lack of tradition, there is a limited number of psychological treatments that are prop-erly validated by controlled clinical trial that includes a large enough sample, a prospective design, an adequate control group, randomized assignment of groups, blind evaluation of results and a medium- to long-term follow-up of patients. To make matters worse, some studies that have a good part, if not all, of these features use very indirect measurements of effectiveness that do not make it possible to show that a specific psychological treatment significantly reduces one type of symptoms, the number of hospitalizations, etc. And in reality, strictly speaking that is really the only thing that should be important to us, at least in principle, as therapists. This does not mean that an improve-ment in certain non-nuclear aspects of the disorder is not important: it is, but at a level immediately below symptomatic improvement, and therefore two levels below the primary objective ("curing" the disorder, somewhat utopian for more than 90% of psychiatric disorders). Fortunately, thanks to a number of studies that will be reviewed throughout this manual, the usefulness of psy-choeducation in improving the course of bipolar patients has been able to be determined, and currently we are able to go to a second level in which we examine what other improvements are obtained with psychoeducation, apart from the most obvious, which is a reduction in the number of episodes and hospitalizations.

The implementation of psychoeducation therefore involves a number of advantages for the treatment of bipolar patients, in addition to those that obviously result from its prophylactic effectiveness. In the first place, the principal advantage of long-duration group psychoeducation treatment is the improvement in the quality of care perceived by our patients, which frequently results in improved therapeutic alliance and pharmacological adherence and in a better ability of the patient to ask for help in complex situations, such as autolytic ideation, or in some cases susceptibility and self-referentiality characteristic of the beginning of some manic episodes. The increased frequency of visits and the incorporation of other professionals, in addition to psychiatry, helps patients feel that they have an active part to play in their treatment, integrated into the team of people in charge of carrying out the treatment. Far from jeopardizing the therapeutic relationship between patient and psychiatrist, the incorporation of psychoeducative psychologists, active hospital involvement in the follow-up of the psychoeducation group and the incorporation of a young resident in psychiatry, for example, to provide specific sessions in the psychoeducation program often conveys to patients the idea that there is a whole team of people working to achieve their improvement. On the one hand, this minimizes their fears of not receiving the best treatment available, and on the other hand, prevents some problems characteristic of the therapeutic relationship, problems such as irritability or lack of trust that often arise from the psychopathology itself, which can be an obstacle to receiving proper treatment.

One of our patients, for example, was extremely reticent to tell the psychiatrist any attitude that could suggest the presence of psychotic symptoms. This was the result of the fact that in his first manic episode, with openly delirious symptomatology, the psychiatrist had to proceed with involuntary hospitalization. The patient was then convinced that talking about those symptoms could result in hospitalization, and carefully tended to avoid telling his psychiatrist any thoughts that he believed could be interpreted as psychotic. This resulted in a problem for his treatment. After his participation in the psychoeducation group, the patient learned the importance of the early detection of the warning symptoms of mania, which in his case included – according to his own list – "lack of trust" to avoid hospitalization. He often also used to comment on any attitude of suspicion or mistrust in the follow-up visits with the psychologist, and between the two of them they would decide up to what point this was pathological or not and whether or not it should be mentioned to the psychiatrist. In this way he improved the early detection of his manic episodes, and over time the patient was no longer afraid to tell his psychiatrist about his thoughts of lack of trust.

Psychoeducation specifically eschews the old paradigm of psychiatric and psychological interventions where there has usually existed an excess of "personal touch," based classically on undetermined aspects such as the inspiration and charisma of the therapist. These aspects are absolutely out of any criterion of falsability or scientific rigor. Psychoeducation avoids the pathogenic model of relationship between a "healing" physician and a passive patient. Instead, it provides an appropriate therapeutic alliance based on collaboration, information and trust.

Incomprehension is an opportunistic illness that exacerbates the course of psychiatric disorders, because the uneasiness caused by the symptoms of the disorder is added to the uneasiness resulting from not being understood by others, and what is worse, not understanding what is happening to oneself nor what to expect. Patients who do not know their disorder do not know their lives and feel incapable of making plans or of looking ahead. In the words of one of our patients, he feels "absolutely helpless before the difficult whims of my mood." Psychoeducation cures incomprehension, at least patients' possible incomprehension about what is happening to them. This, doubtless, is crucial to achieving a certain psychological well-being and a better quality of life. A psychoeducated patient ceases feeling guilty and instead feels responsible. This step is the beginning of accepting the need for treatment. It is not rare for our patients, after finishing a group, to tell us that "now at least I understand why," or "now I know what's happening to me and what can happen to me, and contrary to what I used to think, I am no longer frightened – quite the opposite." An interesting phenomenon that occurs during psychoeducation is that, as the psychoeducation sessions progress and the patient understands their disorder, they have the growing sensation of being understood. It should be taken into account that we healthcare professionals are used not to providing too much information to our patients, beyond the therapeutic indications themselves. This often contributes to their having the sensation that we really do not understand what is happening to them, more so still when we remember that they usually do not know, in principle, that we are prescribing one specific drug and not another precisely because we *do understand* what is happening to them. Patients included in a psychoeducation group, on the other hand, are able to sense from our explanations about their disorder that psychiatry has already described and understood situations that they may be living through with shame, isolation or convinced that they are unique and non-transferable. The psychoeducated patient "knows that we know" and that results in an improvement in the therapeutic relationship. Consequently, psychoeducation meets a fundamental right of the patient and of any human being: the right to information.

Another clear advantage of implementing a relatively long psychoeducation program like the one introduced in this manual is the certainty that for at least 6 months, the patient will receive exhaustive treatment, and in all probability this will result in improved emotional stability. It is well known that in the case of bipolar patients the immediately preceding course is the best prognostic indicator of the immediately subsequent course, so ensuring at least 6 months of stability for some patients has the effect of putting them on track, namely "tracking," and clearly improves the subsequent course. Some patients do not benefit so much from the information received in the group and the interaction with the therapists and the rest of the participants as from the effect the treatment has of putting them on track: for at least half a year ensuring adherence, improving habits and abstinence from toxic substances in a bipolar patient is enough, in some cases, to ensure at least another half a year of stability due to the effect of inertia, even though some of the lessons learned during group time are not maintained.

Moreover, the factors that explain the *immediate* improvement of some patients after their incorporation in the group go beyond what they learn about the disorder, managing symptoms or therapeutic adherence. The perception of a weekly follow-up itself helps patients feel more secure when faced with specific stressors, pay more attention to state of mind or remember more often the need to be more regular in sleep.

Furthermore, providing detailed information to the patient about their disorder goes beyond being a simple technique to improve adherence or common sense. Rather, it becomes an act that is nearly essential in the doctor–patient relationship. The time that a doctor dedicates to this activity will obviously be in accordance with the total time available for each visit, ability to convey their knowledge (not always the wisest doctors have the best teaching ability), the complexity of the disorder and the potential role the patient may develop in their own treatment. It would not be very useful, for example, to explain colon cancer in detail because the patient's level of potential involvement is not very high; however, this does not exempt the doctor from the duty of explaining to a patient what is happening to him or her if the patient really wants to know it. On the other hand, educating patients about their disorder is essential for treating illnesses like asthma, diabetes or high blood pressure. Why? Because the patient's behavior such as diet, habits and attitude toward symptoms can be decisive in the course of the illness. Just as it would be absurd to establish a treatment for a diabetic without psychoeducation, we believe treatment of a bipolar disorder without psychoeducation is inappropriate.

# Mechanisms of action of psychoeducation

The final objective of any treatment should be a reduction of symptoms or an improvement in the course of a specific illness. In the case of bipolar disorders, the objective of any maintenance treatment is a reduction in the number of episodes of both polarities and their severity, and as a result, a reduction in the number of hospitalizations. This is true both for pharmacological treatments as well as psychological treatment. The commonplace distinction in which psycho-pharmacology treats symptoms while psychotherapy treats problems is absurd. In clinical psychology, psychological treatment is useful if it improves the course of an illness.

The action mechanisms of psychoeducation can be broken down into three levels (Table 1). At the first level we find those basic mechanisms that comprise partial objectives *per se*, those mechanisms whose lack of fulfillment leads us to say simply that psychoeducation has not worked. They include providing the patient with an adequate awareness of disorder (and also of episode, when necessary), improving pharmacological adherence and facilitating early detection of new episodes. Taken separately, these three partial objectives have been the goal of various programs similar to ours, but we believe that it is the combination of the three that makes our program a solid approach, with high rates of efficacy, even at the cost of being a long treatment. The three basic mechanisms are probably those that are most able to explain the good results of our program, although curiously they are not the ones the patients usually mention as the most relevant ones after completing a group.

At a second level we place the second-order mechanisms, that is, desirable partial objectives that are nevertheless not the exclusive responsibility of the psychoeducation program. At the third level we can place desirable objectives that are considered part of an "excellent scenario," which are to be achieved once the previous levels have been covered. The prevention of suicidal

**Table 1.** Levels and objectives of the action mechanisms of psychoeducation

*Psychoeducation groups: elemental mechanisms (first-level partial objectives)*
- Awareness of disorder
- Early detection of warning symptoms
- Adherence with treatment

*Psychoeducation groups: secondary mechanisms (second-level partial objectives)*
- Controlling stress
- Avoiding substance use and abuse
- Achieving regularity in lifestyle
- Preventing suicidal behavior

*Psychoeducation groups: objectives that are desirable or of therapeutic excellence*
- Increasing knowledge and facing the psycho-social consequences of past and future episodes
- Improving social and interpersonal activity between episodes
- Confronting residual sub-syndromic symptoms and impairment
- Increasing well-being and improving the quality of life

behavior for obvious reasons would be a fundamental objective of any psychiatric treatment, since the ultimate reason for any medical act should be to preserve life. In spite of that, we did not include it as a first-level objective simply because it is not an exclusive objective of psychoeducation or a subject to which too much time is dedicated during the program (generally one session – see p. 89). However, it is an objective that is always present in any approach of our overall treatment program, whether psychological, psychiatric or infirmary. Confronting stress and increasing regularity of habits are also partial second-level objectives. Our approach does not consist explicitly in a set of techniques for controlling anxiety, although we can teach some very specific techniques if we believe that the majority of the group can benefit from them. Regularity of habits is a mechanism of action of our program that also has been fully worked out as an objective by other types of psychological approaches, such as the interpersonal and social rhythm therapy developed by Prof. Frank's group in Pittsburgh. Our program also affects this point and expressly dedicates a session to it (see p. 182), although actually this is a subject that is present from the beginning and throughout the whole program. Practically, in every session one of the co-therapists or even a patient comments on the importance of hours of sleep and regularity of habits. Avoiding the consumption of toxics would be an elemental mechanism in a specific type of population. It is not necessary to work with dual patients to include the subject of avoiding the use and abuse of toxic substances – the reader should note that these substances include not only illegal street drugs and alcohol, but also "everyday products" such as caffeine – which usually have a devastating effect on the course of bipolar disorder.

Thus, it is important to stratify the partial objectives in order to make it very clear whether or not our treatment is effective in a specific patient. A patient with whom we have succeeded in "increasing knowledge and confronting the psychosocial consequences of past and future episodes," but with whom we have failed to try to achieve better adherence with the treatment is a patient for whom we can say that psychoeducation does not work, simply because it will be difficult to reduce the number of episodes and hospitalizations as only a third-level objective is covered. However, covering all first- and second-level partial objectives does indeed guarantee an improvement of the course.

If we review the list of action mechanisms in psychoeducation treatment we can verify that none of them refers to changes in character or temperamental characteristics. This should not surprise the reader, because it should be taken into account that our psychoeducation program starts from a medical and bio-psycho-social model of the disorder based exclusively on the scientific evidence, and this does not tell us that there is any variable related to the personality or intrapsychic conflict – whatever this means – that affects the course of bipolar disorders. For us it is important to mention this explicitly to our patients, both in the initial interview as well as in the first group session. That way we do not create any false expectations or generate unfounded fears. Both of these things, expectations and fears, are very common when the psychiatrist invites the patient to participate in "group therapy," because most of our patients imagine that they are going to be enrolled in some spectacular, dynamic-oriented group where the dramatization of their emotions will take place, or in some type of humanistic group that has cathartic purposes and tendency toward multiple hugs. It is our obligation to refute both assumptions, with the result in some cases of losing a good part of our patients and calming the rest. We prefer to have the psychiatrist who invites the patient to participate in some "lessons on your disorder," since that presentation emphasizes the importance of information, which is the real mechanism of overall action from psychoeducation. Later we will see what the most suitable forms are for presenting the treatment to patients, both by the psychiatrist as well as the psychoeducator.

# Integrating psychoeducation in clinical practice

One of the greatest problems of evidence-based medicine is the distance that often separates tested approaches and suitable approaches. Most clinical trials of a drug can be criticized because they suffer from a certain sample bias (only cooperating patients are included, the frequency of visits is increased, etc.), a bias that is used as an argument against the possibility of generalizing the results of studies. However, although the legitimacy of such criticisms must be recognized, randomized clinical trials are certainly the only method of demonstrating the efficacy of a specific treatment. In real world practice, open series and naturalistic studies can be very useful in determining the applicability and efficiency of a treatment, but not its efficacy, since by definition its methodology is less rigorous. In spite of that, a hierarchically arranged combination of these two strategies is the only way to provide an overall evaluation of the clinical usefulness of any treatment: first the randomized-controlled study is performed, and then, if the results are positive, the open series.

Curiously, the path followed in the field of psychoeducation in bipolar disorders has been exactly the reverse: during the 1970s, 1980s and beginning of the 1990s there were numerous open series articles, hindered by several methodological pitfalls, intended to determine the applicability of a specific program. It was not until the end of the 1990s and the beginning of this century that the first controlled studies on efficacy appeared (Perry et al., 1999; Colom et al., 2003a, b). These studies have made it possible to confirm with certainty something that seems common sense (and to show what is perceived intuitively as being obvious not only is not redundant but is an intrinsic necessity of science), that is, the close relationship between the knowledge a patient has about their pathology and an improvement in its course, an axiom applicable to psychiatric disorders and to the rest of medical disorders. In the case of diabetes, for example, it is often very useful, or practically decisive, that recently diagnosed patients participate in psychoeducation workshops in which their disorder is explained to them – what diet and behavioral habits are recommended, how they should check their blood sugar level and how to inject themselves with insulin. Something similar occurs with some cardiovascular pathologies, as well as with asthma. In the case of bipolar disorders, a pathology that is complex from the clinical and conceptual point of view as well as from the perspective of its treatment, it would seem impossible for a recently diagnosed patient to be able to acquire, practically by infused science, enough knowledge of their disorder to allow them optimal management of it. This makes it even more necessary to implement psychoeducation in the treatment algorithms of the bipolar patient. Moreover, a psychoeducation program is essential within the context of public health, where the limited time available for medical examinations in most cases makes it difficult for the psychiatrist to carry out the necessary educative work. Not infrequently, therefore, time constraints may convert the rich doctor–patient relationship into a brief meeting between prescriber and consumer of psychotropic drugs, with no time for the educational component. A psychoeducation group is an efficacious and cost-efficient (i.e. useful and economical) way of complementing pharmacological treatment and providing the patient with the necessary knowledge to manage the disorder. But more than anything else, going beyond a structured program within an integral, multidisciplinary therapeutic approach, psychoeducation should be an attitude of the doctor toward the patient, an attitude that involves educating patients about their disorder and informing them about the drugs, as well as closely monitoring the symptomatology.

The program that this book presents (Table 2) is a long, exhaustive program of proven efficacy designed to be delivered by qualified professionals. We know that there is a wide variety of logistical limitations, from not having an appropriate room for the treatment to not having trained psychologists, as well as the problem of adherence with the group's schedules by many patients. Such difficulties as these can prevent the incorporation of this program into the normal clinical practice. In any case, it would be possible to work with reduced psychoeducation programs, although it is still yet to be shown that they can achieve an effectiveness similar to a program of 21 sessions. Table 3 shows an example of a reduced program we are using, experimentally, in Barcelona. Setting aside

**Table 2.** Sessions of the Barcelona psychoeducation program for bipolar disorders

---

Session 1.  Introduction: Presentation and rules of the group

*Unit 1. Awareness of the disorder*
Session 2.  What is bipolar disorder?
Session 3.  Etiological and triggering factors (causes)
Session 4.  Symptoms I: Mania and hypomania
Session 5.  Symptoms II: Depression and mixed episodes
Session 6.  Evolution and prognosis

*Unit 2. Drug adherence*
Session 7.  Treatment I: Mood stabilizers
Session 8.  Treatment II: Antimanic drugs
Session 9.  Treatment III: Antidepressants
Session 10. Plasma levels of mood stabilizers: lithium, carbamazepine and valproate
Session 11. Pregnancy and genetic advice
Session 12. Psychopharmacology vs. alternative therapies
Session 13. Risks associated with interruption of the treatment

*Unit 3. Avoiding substance abuse*
Session 14. Psychoactive substances: risks in bipolar disorder

*Unit 4. Early detection of new episodes*
Session 15. Early detection of mania and hypomanic episodes
Session 16. Early detection of depressive and mixed episodes
Session 17. What to do when a new phase is detected?

*Unit 5. Regular habits and stress management*
Session 18. Regularity of habits
Session 19. Stress-control techniques
Session 20. Problem-solving strategies
Session 21. Final session

---

an aspect that really cannot be set aside, that the 6-month treatment has been properly tested and short psychoeducation programs still have not, working with a long program has a number of potential disadvantages, but also a number of advantages. Among the disadvantages we can include:

1  Foreseeably, a group in a long program will have a greater *number of dropouts* (i.e. patients who will stop attending sessions before the end of

**Table 3.** Sessions for a reduced version of the psychoeducation program for bipolar patients

Session 1. Concept and causes
Session 2. Symptoms I: Mania and hypomania
Session 3. Symptoms II: Depression and mixed conditions
Session 4. Evolution and prognosis
Session 5. Mood stabilizers
Session 6. Antimanic drugs and antidepressants
Session 7. Learning to detect episodes
Session 8. What to do when there is decompensation?

the program). They will therefore not obtain much benefit from being included. Our studies show a dropout percentage of close to 25%, a figure similar to the dropout rate of other shorter psychological treatments; in our pilot studies with short treatments we obtained similar percentages.

2  The *economic expense* that a 6-month treatment could involve is greater, but this point is easily refuted if we consider the savings represented by the reduction in the number of hospitalizations and relapses facilitated by this treatment, something the short treatments have yet to demonstrate.

However, there are many advantages to working with a program of long duration:

1  *Content*: A 6-month program allows many interesting subjects to be approached, without overlooking practically any relevant aspect or take any aspect for granted, an error that often occurs in short groups.

2  *Participation*: The 6-month program allows greater participation of the patients, which in turn contributes decisively to an improvement in learning the content, in the dynamics of the group and in adherence with the psychoeducation treatment itself, and probably to reducing the stigma and feeling of isolation.

3  *Cohesion*: Twenty-one weeks of contact allow the group to be strongly cohesive, among other things, and the patients to feel trusting enough to ask questions or make comments that perhaps they would not do in other contexts. The simple fact of knowing other people who suffer from bipolar disorder and being able to share experiences for 6 months is often very positive in overcoming a life of isolation and stigma that bipolar

patients often suffer, which is frequently manifested in phrases like "I'm really weird," "no one suffers like I do" or "no one can understand what I've been through."

4 *Modeling*: The frequent contact with the other members of the group facilitates the patients exercising a "modeling" effect among themselves, that is, each of them learns from the errors of the others, or incorporates in their repertory healthy behavior of other members of the group. In a group for a program of short duration, it is difficult for patients to reach this level of learning from each other. During the 6 months that the group lasts, it often happens that some of our patients suffer a relapse, which allows the rest to learn from the errors of others (e.g. patients who say during a session that they want to stop the pharmacological treatment and after 2 weeks suffer a relapse, or patients who boast about consuming toxics, etc.). Obviously, this type of modeling was not designed *a priori* – that would clearly be contrary to professional ethics – but it certainly represents an enormous practical advantage. On many occasions we have the impression that pharmacological adherence improves in greater measure after a patient witnesses the relapse of a non-compliant fellow member than after attending five theoretical sessions about the advantages of the medication.

5 *Tracking*: One of the best predictors of a good prognosis for bipolar disorders is without a doubt the immediately preceding course; that is, the patient's clinical course in the last year helps us predict the course during the next year. It is difficult in just 6 months to stabilize a patient with a clinical history of constant cycling, among other things because of a question of cycling inertia. On the other hand, the more time a patient is euthymic, the less probability there will be of a relapse, although this probability will never be zero. Thus, a long program of psychoeducation that ensures good pharmacological adherence, appropriate managing of symptoms, regular habits and which avoids the consumption of toxics, at least during the 6 months that the treatment lasts, also ensures in many cases that a patient remains euthymic during that same period, even though this is due simply to the frequency of the visits, to the commitment with the therapist and the other members of the group, or to other factors that in principle are not part of the psychoeducation itself. In short, psychoeducation treatment of long duration has an orienting

effect on many patients, so that the probability that those patients remain euthymic will be greater at least for 6 months, which in turn will have a positive effect on the course of their disorder for at least the next 6 months.

For these reasons, although we understand the logistical need to reduce the number of sessions of the program, we continue to believe firmly in the greater effectiveness of the long programs which, in spite of being more costly, have obvious added advantages.

Another question we are often asked is why carry out the psychoeducation in a group. The answer is very simple: because the advantages of this format are far greater than its disadvantages. The only disadvantage we can think of has to do with the apparent lack of confidentiality, something that most patients do not see as a shortcoming because they feel they are surrounded by people who suffer from the same disorder and in a safe place, where they can freely express their fears and anxieties. Moreover, the advantages of working in a group are obvious:

1  It allows modeling.
2  It facilitates the support of patients among themselves.
3  It reduces the stigma.
4  It facilitates the awareness of the disorder.
5  It increases the social network of the patients.
6  It is more efficient (i.e. more economical).

# When to introduce psychoeducation?

Introducing a psychological treatment can represent a great advance in the treatment of our patients, or a resounding failure with regrettable consequences, especially if it is the first time we try such a strategy. In the same way poor pharmacological adherence presented by some bipolar or schizophrenic patients can be explained, in some cases, by the unhappy experiences from the side effects suffered the first time they took antipsychotic drugs. For example, the first contact between a patient and a psychological treatment can be crucial in explaining the subsequent response to treatment. We are not now going to digress into mysteries of other paradigms about whether or not to shake hands with our patients and look them in the eye. In principle, they are your hands, your patients and your eyes, so do whatever common sense tells you. We, the authors of this book, are polite and we shake hands with someone when we greet them, and in principle we see no problem with looking anyone in the face. Moreover, we have enough assertiveness to maintain a suitable visual contact with our patients. When we refer to the first contact with the patient, we mean the moment when the psychological approach is introduced and the way in which it is presented to the patient.

If we limit ourselves to psychoeducation, it is completely reasonable to begin treatment when the patient is euthymic. A manic patient should absolutely not be introduced into a psychoeducation group. First, because the behavioral alterations peculiar to the mania could cause serious problems to the coexistence of the group and seriously alter group functioning. Furthermore, the distractability, the tachypsychia and the other cognitive alterations of a manic patient would make it difficult for the patient to benefit from the treatment. This does not mean some psychoeducative concept cannot be included with positive results during a hospitalization, in a one-on-one setting, as is already done in most cases, but we believe that a long, structured approach makes no sense. What is more, the patient may experience contact with the psychologist as being extremely awkward – and, in fact, it would really be awkward because at least one of the two parts would be presenting severe behavioral and cognitive problems and some weeks later patients may not remember that it was they that had those difficulties – which could hinder incorporation into a psychoeducation group when they are euthymic.

If patients are incorporated in the group when they are euthymic and then become manic during the group, we should exclude them from the group and give them the opportunity to be incorporated in another one after they have recovered their mood stability. Our experience has shown us that, although this is obviously undesirable, the rest of the patients often learn a great deal about mania if one of their group fellows becomes manic during the program. The patients understand, for example, that the behavioral alterations peculiar to the mania are quite objectifiable, easily perceived by others but often not considered pathological by the person suffering from them. They can also learn that many times irritability is a genuine part of the mania and not a personality feature, and understand that awareness of disorder undergoes serious alterations during mania. Patients can clearly understand that a condition they experience as non-pathological can be seen by others as quite garish and unhealthy.

One of our patients, whom we will call "H," came to one of the sessions after a couple of weeks of absence. His appearance was somewhat disheveled and he was clearly nervous during the time preceding the start of the session. When we began the session we invited the participants, as usual, to talk about everything that seemed relevant to them in relation to their disorder in recent days. H abruptly interrupted the therapist and after a somewhat confused and grandiloquent speech about his disorder being sort of a gift, offered to take over as therapist from that time on, since, according to his words, he had been ill but no longer was and he wanted to teach the others in the group how to recover their health without the need to take any medication. The therapists allowed H to speak for 5–10 min because, on the one hand, we thought that interrupting him could result in violence, and on the other hand, H's symptomatology would allow us to explain to the others the manic phase without too much difficulty, since H was performing as an authentic model of mania and that could be very beneficial for the rest of the group. After that time we politely interrupted H and asked the group for feedback. They all agreed, using phrases like "you're a bit high," "I experienced something very similar and ended up awful" or "you're not like that, I think you're sick." As would be expected, H did not react very well to these comments, accusing his co-members of being "blind sheep." One of the co-therapists convinced H to "discuss this separately because it seems as though the group does not understand you." The duty psychiatrist decided that H should be hospitalized because he was suffering from a mania with psychotic symptoms. The group understood this hospitalization as the last step in H's manic ascent. No one in the group reacted with hostility toward H, even though he had been disrespectful to them; on the contrary, they all reacted positively, recognized what happened as a manic episode and something to be avoided, and some of them visited H during his hospitalization.

With regard to hypomania, in principle we would not recommend to include any hypomanic patient since the jocularity, distractability and facility for arguing are elements that are usually not helpful in providing group solidarity. Moreover, hypomania is characteristically unstable and frequently the prelude to a complete manic episode. Nevertheless, in the case of euthymic patients who become hypomanic during the group program, we can be much more flexible because in most cases they can be self-limiting by following the lessons acquired during the sessions, and the group itself can be used to point out the pathological aspects of the condition. Most patients who have already spent time in the group are much more open to an observation from another patient about his disorder than a contribution of the same kind by the psychiatrist or psychologist. It is therefore not unusual for us to allow hypomanic patients to continue in the group as long as their behavior is not too disruptive. These patients can serve as an illness model for the others and the group may help them to deal with their symptoms.

With respect to mixed phases, in general, it is not advisable to include or try to keep in the group a patient who initiates mixed symptoms, among other things because the patient nearly always explicitly rejects going to the group. In any event, the predominant symptoms in most mixed episodes (i.e. irritability, anxiety, negative thoughts, tachypsychia) would not facilitate adaptation to the treatment.

The handling of depressive or negative cognitions, which also appear in some euthymic patients, is extremely delicate during a group psychoeducation session, because having the patients begin to sympathize with such cognitions must be avoided, especially those that have to do with the disorder ("we're a bunch of losers," "what lousy luck – we'd be better off dead," "we'll never do anything good," etc.). If this occurs, the therapists must explicitly ally themselves with the most optimistic sector of the group, provided there is one, for two reasons. Confronting the thoughts of one patient with those of another produces good results and we avoid the addendum of "sure, it's easy to be optimistic when you are not suffering from the disorder." It is also helpful that we openly support patients who resist pessimism to prevent them from becoming prisoners of fear, or begin to entertain negative ideas about the disorder, which in most cases will cause the patient not to return to the group because "I left worse than when I went in."

Seriously depressed patients should not be included in a psychoeducational group, among other things because they would not get sufficient benefit because of their own cognitive alterations in that phase (slowness, attention and memory difficulties). Moreover, there is a risk of worsening the situation and accentuating the hopelessness, because a depressed patient easily takes the most negative part of the information provided by the therapist. If a patient included in the psychoeducation program suddenly suffers a serious major depressive episode, we would suggest him to be excluded from the group and be offered the possibility of continuing with an individual psychological follow-up to avoid the feeling of abandonment and to control autolytic ideation, in addition to the possibility of being incorporated in psychoeducative groups later.

How should we handle psychotic symptoms in a group? In principle, the presence of psychotic symptoms in a patient justifies exclusion. Under no circumstances should we try to apply some type of cognitive approach to those symptoms. Setting aside the more than arguable usefulness of such a strategy, which to date has not been shown to be effective in a controlled study, it is possible that the fact that this approach is carried out in front of the whole group could be a negative experience for the patient, since he may think – not without reason – that we are exposing him to the other members. The recommended approach is for one of the co-therapists to accompany psychotic patients to a separate office, and with their cooperation, attempt to analyze to what extent the patients themselves interpret specific thoughts as psychotic. In any case, if none of the co-therapists is a psychiatrist, we should immediately contact a psychiatrist to have the pharmacological prescription changed if necessary. With respect to the attitude we should take before the rest of the group concerning delirious symptomatology in one of their members, once that patient has been removed, the most appropriate method is to try to review the psychotic symptoms and to locate that symptomatology in the disorder while explicitly avoiding compassion, criticism, ridicule or laughing, which are all very common reactions to the psychotic symptoms of others.

# Formal aspects of the psychoeducation program

## Number and type of patients

The ideal size of a psychoeducation group is between 8 and 12 patients. It is possible to work with fewer than 8 participants, but this can reduce the wealth of the patients' contributions and opportunities to interact. Working with more patients can often be very uncomfortable for the therapists as well as for the patients, because they can think that the therapists are not paying enough attention or that, because of time restrictions, they do not have enough time to take part in the roundtable discussion. Furthermore, it is very difficult to develop a feeling of belonging to a group if it is too large. This often results in poor adherence with the group's schedules as well as with the rest of the rules, and in general, poor involvement of the patients. Since the dropout rate is around 25%, we have observed that it is useful to start the group with 15 or 16 patients, which ends up being reduced to 10–12 after the first four or five sessions. However, if we start with about 10 patients, as we had done in the pilot groups prior to the clinical trial, we can end up with more than 25% dropouts, because the patients do not want to join a group with fewer than 8 participants. Thus, in one of the groups we ended up working with only four subjects.

To date we have not been able to find a good dropout predictor, but patients with a comorbid personality disorder or substance abuse certainly are not as compliant, as often happens with any type of pharmacological or psychological treatment.

We always attempt to have the groups balanced with regard to gender. With respect to age, the idea is to have the group homogeneous enough to generate a communal feeling but sufficiently heterogeneous so as not to lose the value it represents for many young patients to know someone who has the same disorder but "has done well in life" (in the words of a young patient about an older patient). Older patients in turn generally accept the role of veterans and see reflected in the younger patients some of their past attitudes, something they also evaluate as positive. In any event, in our group we establish an age limit of at least 18 due to the characteristics of the center itself (we only provide psychiatric care to adults), while we set the upper limit at 55. Patients older than 55 can be included in a senior psychoeducation program that is shorter than the standard one. This is a program that focuses more on some of the aspects that concern patients of that age group (drug interactions of psychotropics, contraindications of psychotropics with respect to other medical illnesses, cognitive deterioration), and in which we mostly ignore other aspects that we have determined are less problematic for these patients: we drop the session on bipolar disorder and pregnancy for obvious reasons, nor do we include any sessions on stimulants and other psychoactives to which, in principle, patients in this age group do not have easy access. However, we do talk about alcohol because this is a highly prevalent problem in this age group.

We do not establish any distinction between patients with bipolar disorder I or II, but from the outset we clearly explain the difference between the two subtypes. For research purposes, it would be interesting to be able to establish if psychoeducation has the same effect on one subtype as on the other.

With regard to friendships among the participants in the group, we do not encourage them, but we also do not prohibit them. Some groups acquired the habit of going for a coffee half an hour before the session or immediately after, and appear to have continued talking very openly about the disorder. According to one of the patients, "In the café is where we really did the therapy and where more things came out." Other participants even organized dinners over time. To our knowledge, of more than 200 patients that have participated in the psychoeducation program quite a number of friendships were established. Obviously this is not the objective of the program, but it is completely understandable if we take into account that the network of social relationships of many bipolar patients has declined a great deal due to the disorder.

With regard to pairing off or love affairs between members of the group, it is not unusual for some members to begin a love relationship, again due, in part, to the limited social network of some of our patients. We should emphasize that, in every case in which this has happened, we therapists found out long after the sessions ended, so that the relationship does not appear to have interfered in any way with the functioning of the group. The only problem related to love interest we have had in nearly 10 years of experience in working with groups involved a bipolar patient with a borderline personality disorder who developed an erotomania toward one of the group's participants, with serious behavioral alterations that could have been annoying for her and were interfering in the psychoeducation program. We therefore felt obligated to exclude that patient and offer him the possibility of joining the next group.

## The therapists

It is advisable for the group to be directed by more than one therapist. We usually work with one therapist and two co-therapists, who are usually graduates in training. The psychoeducation program can be given by a psychologist or psychiatrist, but in either case it is essential to have enough experience in handling groups and in the treatment of bipolar disorders.

## Materials required

Psychoeducation is without doubt a very efficient treatment. Aside from its indisputable efficacy, it should be remembered that it is really an inexpensive treatment among other things because no extra materials are required to implement it: all that is needed is a room prepared to accommodate a group of between 15 and 20 people. We also use a chalkboard where we note the most relevant information of each session, draw course graphs, etc.

In each session we distribute teaching materials comprised of two or three sheets that summarize what is explained during the session. Most of our patients consider these materials to be very useful as a reminder, and they all ask us for them when they have not been able to attend a session. We have even observed that some patients use them to psychoeducate their families, because they encourage them to read them after the session and then they talk about the materials with them. Although this is not something we expressly tell our patients to do, and in spite of the fact that we are aware of the risks of this type of action (although it is in written form, the information can be distorted to a astonishing degree) and we have set up a parallel program designed specifically for family members of the patients. We believe that this practice can help to establish the information and sometimes result in a first contact between the family of our patients and the medical model of the bipolar disorder.

As can be seen in this volume, the material for the sessions is written in a language that is simple and accessible to anyone with no training in psychiatry or psychology, and is respectful yet clear and forceful in its assertions.

When we started our psychoeducation program we usually assigned homework. As a result of the low rate of response by our patients, in recent groups we have abandoned that strategy, even though we believe that it would be useful to many patients as a reminder and help them establish the knowledge.

## Organization of the sessions

These sessions last for 90 min, and should be held weekly. Sessions schedule should enhance adherence to the program for all patients, including those who are employed or studying. Practically all sessions follow the same pattern:

- We consider the first 15–20 min to be a warm-up period. We begin with informal conversation, not necessarily related to the bipolar disorder, talking with the members of the group about the news, for example, always striving to maintain a friendly, sincere tone, not avoiding jokes and without feeling responsible for bearing the weight of the conversation. After a few minutes we can begin to make proposals that concern psychoeducation work *per se*. A first undertaking would be a roundtable discussion, patient by patient, in which we invite them but never force them to comment on whether there had been some relevant incident or change in mood during the last week. If patients mention a variation, we will ask if we can question them about it and will determine to what point it seems pathological to us, or not. If we believe it meets the criteria for some type of episode, or medication is needed, one of the co-therapists will ask the patient to accompany them to a separate room where they will have an in-depth interview with the patient and a psychiatric examination of their condition, or in extreme cases, accompany the patient to our own emergency department if this is considered necessary. During this phase we also invite the patients to ask questions that were pending from the previous session, or questions that have arisen since the last week.
- The next 40 min are dedicated to a pretty interactive lecture on the subject of the session. Although there are concrete educational objectives that

must be covered in each session, the patients are allowed to get involved freely when they think it is necessary, and are even encouraged to do so. In some sessions group exercises, graphics or roundtable discussions are carried out to ensure understanding and participation of all of the patients.

- The last half an hour is dedicated to an open discussion of the subject covered in the session. The therapist encourages the patients to participate, and tries to make sure none of them monopolizes the session.

**Part 3**

# Psychoeducation program: sessions and contents

## Unit 1

# Awareness of the disorder

Unit 1 is fundamental, because its objective is to give the patient the basic information about bipolar disorders. We, the professionals, must not fall into the trap of considering that our patients obviously know all the information concerning the causes and symptoms of the disorder, since most of them ignore the biological, clinical and recurrent nature of their disorder. This unit must always be the first, because it will introduce concepts that will later be absolutely necessary during the group program. For example, we do not believe that it makes sense to carry out the brief intervention merely designed to identify the symptoms early, if we have not first correctly defined what the bipolar disorder is and why its symptoms appear. Consequently, we dedicate a very large number of sessions to this matter (the first five) for two main reasons: (1) on the one hand, because we believe that this is the point that warrants more specific work, as demonstrated by the high rates of lack of illness insight, which are associated to poor adherence, and (2) because, in a way, it is a manner of "refocusing" the patient included in a psychoeducation group in the fundamental aspect of their treatment: its biological nature and the need for drugs.

Quite a large number of patients misunderstand their joining the therapy group as the beginning of their "depsychiatrization" or, in other words, the first step toward becoming medication free, and they so declare in the first session. At least, this is what happened in one of our groups. During the first session, we usually ask the patients to introduce themselves saying their name and, if they wish, to comment on an aspect of their disorder they consider relevant and, lastly, what they expect from their participation in the group. Concretely, in this group, the first patient whose term was to speak said that his objective was "to be capable of controlling the disorder by myself and not need so much medication." Either due to a phenomenon of sympathy or social facilitation, or because this was really what they thought, the two patients that followed him also indicated that they expected, respectively, "to stop taking medication," "not to be hospitalized," and "not to have to take other drugs besides lithium." It is absolutely necessary for the therapist to present, from the beginning of the group sessions, both treatments not as opposed but as complementary, and to make it clear that the medication is absolutely necessary, including writing it on the blackboard if necessary. Otherwise, "an antipsychiatry" type of thinking may immerge among the patience of the group, which if properly controlled, will foster poor adherence behavior: one of our patients used to say that nothing had ever happened to him when he had stopped taking the medication, which was not completely true, because he tended to have mixed and manic results with extreme ease and little awareness of decompensation, and this seemed to have a negative impact on another two patients, one of whom stopped taking part of the medication for a week, thinking that nothing would happen to him.

The fact that we, the psychologists, placed so much emphasis from the beginning on the drug treatment, eliminates from the start to any temptation of "making an opposition group" the idea of which may come to some of our patients.

The sessions on the concept of disorder are extremely interesting to our patients who sometimes react with surprise when placed with certain statements. These are usually the more "open" sessions; in other words, sessions in which the patients are invited more to give their opinion concerning the topic discussed. The purpose of this approach is merely for us to get an idea of which beliefs and attitudes are being handled by our patients in order to find out exactly on what points we must emphasize, and to understand what prejudices they have in connection with the disorder, since they are often dominated by guilt. Certain patients react or explanations with resistance; in this case, the better strategy is to allow the members of the group to discuss between them the contents of the sessions rather than for us to act as defense lawyers for the medical model, since if we do so quite a few patients will accuse us of having corporate-like attitudes. In exchange, if it is another patient that defines the biological character of the bipolar disorder and the need for treatment, the "rebel" patient is left without weighty arguments.

One of the topics that comes up in the sessions of this first unit is the stigma, the social scorn of mental disorders and the way the patients must speak about their diagnosis to their circle. On the later point, we would be extremely cautious, since patients must choose very carefully the people to whom they disclose their disorders and those to whom they do not. If the patient decides to explain it, we recommend the following method:

1  Try to explain the bipolar disorders by focusing in particular on its biological aspects; in other words, starting by its definition as a brain disorder: the bipolar disorder is a disorder that affects the limbic system, neurotransmitters, and the endocrine system. In this case, even though this is an oversimplification, we will avoid any comment about the interaction of these causes with others, of a rather psychological or social nature, because this may cause confusion.

2  Place more emphasis on the medical symptoms (tiredness, fatigue, lost of appetite and sleeping more due to depression, physical unrest, and insomnia for mania and hypomania) rather than on the psychiatric ones, since the latter are usually associated to the black legend they generate in the media. Nobody will be amazed or surprised if you say that, because of a disorder, you had a period when it was difficult for you to leave your bed and you were extremely weak and tired, but everybody will open their eyes wide and may even look at you strangely if you say that you thought that your life was senseless and that you wanted to die. Only a professional or somebody who also experienced a depression may understand that this is a disorder.

3  Avoid discussing the symptoms, which may awake morbid interest in the interlocutor (suicide ideas, hallucinations and delirium, hypersexuality, aggressive episodes, etc.).

4  Following the simple advice, it is hard to go wrong. Anyway, compare the following two statements and choose the one that is more similar to yours:

"I have a mental disorder, which sometimes makes me loose control over my own will. Sometimes I am like crazy, a bit 'round the bend, and they have to hospitalize me in a madhouse and once I tried to kill myself. I take some pills that make me feel sluggish. My neighbor says that these pills may make me dependent and sometimes I believe I am becoming a druggy."

Or:

"I have a disorder that affects various systems in my body, such as the limbic system and the thyroid. Sometimes it has given me trouble (e.g. insomnia, nervousness, and restlessness) and once I even had to be hospitalized. At other times, this disorder takes away all my strength and makes me feel extremely tired, and with several physical discomforts. Fortunately, I am taking medication that helps me a lot, even though it does create some problems."

It is obvious that the best is for your statements to be similar to the latter and not to include any of the former, although both may be explaining the same situation.

Even though this issue is not regulated in any session, it will be very important for the therapist to encourage this debate, since it is a topic that creates anxiety in practically all our patients.

In the fifth session we may teach our patients to make a life chart, provided we do not find that it is too complex. Generally, it is a technique that helps a lot, even though it makes some patients anxious. If we have chosen the life chart, in the following sessions we will invite a couple of patients in each session to present their chart and we will take advantage of the situation to discuss the most significant aspects.

Even though in the beginning we dedicate only the first five sessions to Unit 1 (plus the introduction session), the topic of the awareness of the disorder is fundamental, and will regularly appear in all the sessions of the program.

# Session 1

# Presentation and rules of the group

## Goal

The goal of Session 1 is to take contact with the group and to explain the existing rules to the members. These rules are basic for the good functioning of the group, and are also intended to create a good environment that would facilitate patient participation. Although one of the scientific fathers of group treatment, Yalom, openly defines the bipolar patient as "one of the worst calamities that may befall a group," the truth is that our experience indicates quite the contrary. The bipolar patient usually adapts very well to the psychoeducation group, especially if we achieve proper homogeneity/heterogeneity balance among the members concerning age, sex, seriousness, etc. To date, there are many patients who have become perfectly integrated in the functioning of the group, taking a participative role and being extremely collaborative and respectful to the other group members and the therapist. This is not at all strange: our patients correctly integrate in the group because they understand immediately that they may get great benefits from the experience, that both of them and their disorders will be quickly accepted and understood, and that in the psychoeducation program the aspects of great interest to them are being worked on. This is something that probably did not happen in Yalom's groups.

## Procedure

- Before starting the session, we will prepare the room by placing several chairs in a circle and, slightly distanced from the others, as many chairs as there are therapists by the blackboard.
- In general, the patients wait in the waiting room of the center. One of the co-therapists will go and bring them in from the waiting room, so that they all enter the group room together.

- We will greet the patients naturally, if this is our style. If our usual style is not to be natural, we will seriously think of changing our job.
- After stating our name and profession, the first step is to present the program, its objectives, its duration (21 sessions lasting 90 min each), and the methods we will use. We will also explain "what a psychoeducation program *is not*," in other words that a psychoeducation program is not an intervention designed to tackle childhood problems or traumas, to make them "put their emotions on the table," to discuss intrapsychological conflicts or merely to share experiences.
- Next, we will explain in detail the rules of the group. We will warn them that failing to respect some of these rules may lead to the expulsion of a patient from the psychoeducation program. The rules are as follows:
  - *Confidentiality*: The patients must not discuss outside the group either the identity of the other members or what they say during the sessions. Usually, we explain to our patients that, the same as the psychiatrists and psychologists respect professional secrecy, they must agree to keep secret the identity of the other members of the group. In exchange, we will also make it clear that everything we therapists say, may be freely discussed in public.
  - *Attendance*: Since there is a rather long waiting list to be included in the psychoeducation program, participation in the group is practically a privilege. For this reason, and to facilitate the group sentiment, attendance to all sessions is mandatory. Any patient who fails to attend five sessions will be forced to leave the group. If there is a reason to explain these absences, the patient will be invited to take part in a future group.
  - *Punctuality*: Punctuality is fundamental for the normal course of the sessions. Failing to systematically respect the schedule of the group will lead to the exclusion of the infringing patient.
  - *Respect*: We will explicitly request all members of the group to respect the opinions of their participants even if they do not share them and never to lack respect to the rest of the group either by comments, laughing or attitudes. Repeatedly infringing this rule may lead to exclusion.
  - *Participation*: Intervening in the sessions, in other words posing questions, sharing experiences with the group and advising other participants, is not mandatory but it is highly recommendable in order to best take advantage of the group.

- *Benefit*: It is also not mandatory to do the weekly assignments in writing, if assigned, but we consider that it is the best way of benefiting from the participation in the program.
  - There is *no prohibition related to the meeting* of the patients outside the sessions.
- After explaining the rules in detail, we will start a round of questions, but not before making sure that all the patients have understood and respect the rules presented. If there is a patient who fails to respect the rules from the beginning, which has only happened to us twice, we will invite them to leave the room.

  Next, in a much more relaxed tone, we will introduce ourselves. It is highly recommendable to break the ice and to make the presentations by using some type of games. Any of the classic group dynamic games may be useful. We will use the following ones:
  - In the *first round*, all the therapists and the patients introduce themselves. The therapists introduce themselves by their name, occupation, and availability. The patients may introduce themselves by their name and, if they wish with "a comment on your life work, hobbies, or desires, not necessarily related to the disorder."
  - After this round, we will do another *remembrance round* of the names. The first patient to the right says their name, the second patient to the right must say their own name and the name of the first patient, the third patient says their own name and the names of the preceding two participants and so forth until the last patient of the circle says the names of the entire group. Then another round begins. If a patient does not remember a name, the person who was forgotten will help them remember. The therapist must also participate in the game.
- After this game, we will end the session, generally with a positive comment such as, "good, by what I have seen besides the fact that we will all learn a lot, we may have a lot of fun," especially if the game was amusing, which it most frequently is. Finally, we will invite the patients to the next session.

## Useful tips

- The first session is crucial to establish good contact between the therapists and the patients. It is important to explain clearly what the group is and what it is not, with basic examples. We, for example, simply explain that "this is not a therapy group as we are used to seeing in Woody Allen movies, nor will we expect a great emotional explosion such as 'I am your father, Joe, I am your father!'" (we play out the last one and so far it has worked very well as a joke).

- In general, we present the psychoeducation program as "a course in which we will teach you what the bipolar is, and certain techniques and tricks to better handle the disorder and also to stay ahead of it."
- In spite of the fact that we, as therapists, feel quite comfortable using humor, the reading of the group rules must be a "serious" moment, since seriousness gives our patients a security in connection with the content of the rules and in addition makes them understand that they are rigorous.
- During the presentation game, the therapists must introduce themselves before the patients, with a simple formula that includes saying their name, title, current occupation in the hospital and – very important – the place and hours during which they may be found. It is also necessary to make it clear to the patients that it does not bother us if they call us or if they call us without an appointment when necessary, and that we work as a team and, therefore, we can give them several names of professionals from the same team whom they may consult. This makes it extremely easy for the patient to take action early in case of a relapse symptom and, in fact, is the first step in establishing an emergency plan, even though this aspect is usually worked on in a more advanced place of the program.

Our presentation, which we include below as an example, must still be adapted to the personal style of each therapist. It is more or less as follows:

"My name is Francesc Colom and I am a clinical psychologist. I work in the bipolar disorder program, conducting the psychoeducation groups for 11 years. You can find me from Monday through Friday at such-and-such time, and such-and-such time in the office x. You can also contact me by telephone at the following number (write it on the blackboard and keep it there throughout the session). Among other things, during the sessions we will learn to identify the signs of relapse of bipolar disorders. It does not bother me at all if you call me or come to see me if you have the slightest suspicion of a relapse and, moreover, it is your responsibility as patients. Certain patients hesitate to call me because they believe I am very busy and that it bothers me and it constitutes extra work for me. Of course, I am usually very busy, but I prefer to spend 5 or 10 min talking on the phone with one of you, rather than not being able to talk to you and to have to hospitalize you, let's say, 2 weeks later. This gives us much more work! Among other things, because I am able to speak to you by telephone while I am comfortably seated in my office and, if you get hospitalized, one of us would have to go to the hospitalization room every morning, and this means getting up, going out of the office, and accumulation of visits in the office, etc. So that both for your sake and my own, I hope you will not have to be hospitalized and I prefer it if you call me, no matter if it is a false alarm: I rather attending ten false alarms and catching a single relapse that not catching any relapse at all. If you do not find me, you may try to locate your psychiatrist, Dr. V, or psychologists A, B, and C in offices d, e, and f, or the other psychiatrists on the team, Dr. G, H, and I. Let's face it; they are much less attractive and not as nice as I am, but they will take care of you. All of us are paid to visit patients like you, even though we are paid less than you think, so that it is also our duty to see you. Please be so kind as not to leave us without a job."

The tone may be more or less joking and casual, according to everybody's personal style, but it is important to convey the following messages explicitly:
- What our availability is.
- It is necessary to locate a member of the team when faced with any relapse.
- We do not object to seeing patients without an appointment or to take their calls. The objective is to avoid that the symptoms become more severe.
- We are part of a team, and if we cannot be found it is possible to find one of our colleagues.
- During the presentation, we must make it clear that the act of introducing one's self to the group, like any other act, is voluntary and that each patient must say what they want to say about themselves, provided it is true.

## Patient material

Any human group is governed by a series of rules that facilitate its functioning, prevent conflicting situations that may impair coexistence, and establish response patterns in situations that may interfere with its good functioning. We will not be an exception and for the next 20 weeks therapists and patients will be a group, even though each of us comes from our own position, because we are all in the same boat. Consequently, we need to define the rules of our group, which on the other hand, are common sense rules and will allow all of you to take maximum advantage of your participation. These rules are as follows:

- *Respect*: All the participants in the group must be respectful to the other participants and their opinions, even if you disagree. Consequently, disparaging, mocking, or sarcastic comments about other participants will not be allowed. We may laugh with another participant, and it happens, but we will never laugh at another participant.
- *Confidentiality*: A person's health or a disorder condition is part of their privacy, their private life. Participation in this group implies "confessing" in front of the other member's own diagnosis, in this case the bipolar disorder, so that all the members of the group must respect its confidentiality. Obviously, this group is not a secret club, but its participants are not allowed to disclose the diagnosis of other members to others. In the same way, we are bound by the ethics code of psychiatrists and psychologists to keep secret the identity of our patients and what we know about them, the patients in the group must not comment to outsider people aspects concerning the privacy of other members. On the contrary, everything we, the therapists, may say can be openly discussed with friends family or acquaintances, since this is information about the bipolar disorders and not aspects of our privacy.
- *Attendance*: We are asking the patients to regularly attend all the sessions of the program (20 more after this one). Not doing so would mean, on the one hand, a lack of respect for other patients who are on the waiting list and were unable to join the group and, on the other hand, it would be a serious handicap to understand the information in our program. Any absence must be duly justified for practical reasons, patients cannot continue in the psychoeducation program if they miss five sessions, so that *the fifth absence will cause their exclusion*. If there was a sufficient reason to justify the absence, the patient will be included in subsequent groups.
- *Punctuality*: The sessions of the group will take place every Tuesday from *2 p.m. to 3:30 p.m.*, for example. Coming 10 min late is an accident, coming half an hour late is a lack of respect. Coming late to the sessions interrupts their normal evolution and harms all the participants. Systematically not

respecting the schedule of the group without good reason and without notice will cause the exclusion of the patient.

- *Participation*: The patient decides what degree of involvement he wants. We advise you to actively intervene in the sessions, answering questions, sharing experiences, but you decide. *You do not have to intervene, but it is advisable.*

# What is bipolar disorder?

## Goal

The goal of Session 2 is to introduce patients to the concept of bipolar disorders and to dispel the numerous myths about it, stressing the biological nature of the disorder and attempting to overcome its social stigma.

From the point of view of a hospital-based practice, we tend to think that our own opinion regarding mental illness, in this case bipolar disorder, is probably the one most widely held by society as a whole. Nothing could be further from the truth. Generally speaking, the general public is extremely unaware of the origins and natures of psychiatric disorders. For many of our patients, what we will say in this session is going to be rather surprising. It will revolutionize their lives and change the way they understand their disorder and, consequently, the way they understand themselves as individuals.

Session 2 is often very effective in combating the feelings of guilt that a lot of our patients feel, especially the ones that arise from a strictly psychologistic focus or come directly from dynamic orientation treatments.

## Procedure

- We begin the session, as we always do, with a warm-up phase, where we can simply ask patients how their week was, go over any questions they might have about the guidelines given in Session 1, joke around ("Are you up for this?"), and repeat the name game (see p. 59). This way the mood in the room will be pleasant when we begin the session.
- The session can begin with this statement: "Bipolar disorder results from a change in the mechanisms that regulate mood." This statement can help us establish the biological nature of the disorder. Then, we can begin our session

by making it clear to patients that they can interrupt us whenever a concept is not clear enough to them.

- During the session, we will draw a sketch of the brain on the blackboard and point out the limbic system. This simple gesture, along with comments about it, tends to be very useful for patients to pinpoint the cause of their disorder. Although we, as professionals, could discuss this affirmation – which is, without a doubt, oversimplified here – for endless hours, the statement tends to be crucial for our patients to understand what are not the causes of bipolar disorder and dispel some of the guilt-causing myths that almost always come from paradigms in psychiatry and psychology that are already obsolete or from widely held popular beliefs. Obviously, we must explain to patients that pinpointing the etiology of bipolar disorder in the limbic system is an oversimplification and that during the program we are going to go into the biological aspects of the disorder in more detail.

- In order to introduce the concept of recurrent course, it would be helpful to represent it graphically. We will do it in the following fashion: on the blackboard we will draw two axes – the x-axis, representing time, and the y-axis, representing mood changes (D for more severe depressive episodes, d for mild–moderate depressive symptomatology, E for euthymia, m or H for hypomania, and M for mania). This is, in fact, the presentation of a technique we are going to use often in the program – the mood-chart technique (see p. 101) – so it is a good idea for us to explain it carefully, as many times as necessary, and make sure that everyone understands the meaning of the graph.

- A useful exercise in this session can be to go around the room and ask patients to recall and repeat prejudices and topic sentences that society applies to psychiatric disorders in general ("only weak people have the disorder," "you have to get through it on your own," "it only happens to people who take drugs"). We will write down these phrases on the blackboard and analyze them later. This exercise allows us to, on the one hand, tackle the social stigma weighing on the disorder, but it also lets us see some of the most intimate beliefs our patients have about their disorder, either from the phrases we provide or the ones the rest of the group provides. We can present a list of the "10 Rotten Lies" about bipolar disorders (Table 4) and then discuss them one by one.

**Table 4.** Ten rotten lies about bipolar disorder

| |
|---|
| 1 Doctors made it up. |
| 2 It is a Western-countries' disorder. |
| 3 It is an illness of this century. |
| 4 Only weak people have it. |
| 5 It is a contagious disorder. |
| 6 Psychoanalysis and homeopathy are useful. |
| 7 It is a gift from God. |
| 8 You cause it yourself. |
| 9 It can be controlled without medication. |
| 10 It is an incapacitating disease. |

- The issue involving the disorder's inheritability, which is introduced for the first time in this session, tends to worry our patients, most of all the patients who have children or who want to have them. Since this session does not focus on this issue, we will try to dedicate just a couple of phrases to it, trying most of all not to alarm our patients and suggesting that they talk about it during the session on pregnancy and genetic counseling (see p. 130).
- After questions, we will hand out the material, explain the take-home assignment, and close the session.

## Useful tips

- The general population is very poorly informed about bipolar disorders. Although some of the patients are going to be more or less informed – thanks to books, conferences, Internet searches, talks with their psychiatrist, or through other media – we should keep in mind that it is very likely that most of the members of the group will not have an accurate idea about the disorder they are suffering from. Therefore, we should start at the very beginning, even if some patients complain about this. You should take nothing for granted, because doing so might make some of the patients feel left out from the first few sessions.
- It is important that this session, which is really the first truly informative session, be conducted by the primary therapist. Although other sessions can and should be left to other co-therapists, if the principal therapist is the one directing this session, this tends to make the patient feel that there

is a reference professional with them, and this idea will be very helpful over the course of the program.

- In this session, patients tend to ask why we consider bipolar disorder to be an illness. Our answer should be simple and clear: it is a biological change that has well-described symptoms and that causes people who have it and those around them to suffer.
- Many patients appear eager to receive this information, and this allows them to keep up with the flow of the session and to ask questions that will be discussed in later sessions. We should not lose sight of the goal of this session and should suggest that patients wait until later sessions.
- Some patients ask about the different names for bipolar disorder (bipolar disorder, manic–depressive psychosis, etc.). Although we advocate that they preferably use the term "bipolar disorders," we can briefly comment on the origins of the term "manic–depressive psychosis" and explain why we feel its use is not adequate (it is highly stigmatized socially and, in addition, bipolar disorders do not always require psychotic symptoms or a mania). We should also explain that, in fact, it is a synonym for bipolar disorder and therefore cannot be thought of as a mistaken diagnosis.
- To make our explanation easy to understand, we should always use the example of a thermostat, because it tends to be very useful and patients remember it and explain it to their families, and so we should always present it. The example consists of comparing how a thermostat is useful in a home – you use it to keep the temperature stable, constant and to cause a reaction to changes in the environment – to how the limbic system, which would be the "mood thermostat" in charge of keeping moods stable, constant and react the right way to its surroundings, is useful.
- When we represent the course graphically, we should not draw our representation of periods of euthymia in a perfect straight line, because we want to convey that there are certain highs and lows, although not very pronounced, during euthymia and the mood of a person who does not suffer from bipolar disorder. We usually say that "euthymia is a straight line drawn by a shaky hand, otherwise life would be too boring."
- We prefer to end sessions with a funny, educational story that takes the dramatic feel out of a session's content. In Session 2, we usually tell our patients the story about *The Three Little Bipolar Pigs,* which we use to illustrate to what extent the disorder is biological and also to what extent

our attitude toward it is crucial; otherwise, we could make the group's attitude to be resigned to "no matter what I do, I'm going to have a relapse."
Nonetheless, we admit that the story about *The Three Little Bipolar Pigs*
fits very well in our style as therapists, but if you cannot deal well with the
fine line between the comical and the disrespectful comments, there could
be misunderstandings, so we leave it up to the reader whether or not to
incorporate this story when applying the psychoeducation program. The
story of *The Three Little Bipolar Pigs* goes more or less like this:

"We all know the popular children's tale about the three little pigs who,
when they find out that the big, bad wolf has apparently included them on
his menu without previous consultation, take different preventive measures
with very different results. The first little pig did not take the voracious
wolf's threats very seriously and, despite the warnings and going against all
common sense, thought nothing bad could ever happen to him and that
everything about the wolf was a fairy tale. So he built his house out of straw
and lived in ignorant bliss until the day the wolf came along and with one
puff blew the conceited little pig's shack down, who only became aware of
the danger as he was being digested by the wolf after being properly seasoned, chopped up and roasted. The second little pig only half believed the
wolf was coming. He'd say, "I know there are wolves, but they can't be that
ferocious," so he decided to take some precautions, but not all of the ones
that were at hand – sorry, I mean, at hoof. He built a house out of wood,
which was obviously safer than the one made out of straw, but he decided
not to build it out of a more solid material, because it would have been too
much of a sacrifice. The wolf, against the advice of his doctor, who had
warned him that his cholesterol was through the roof and he had to stop
eating bacon immediately and start exercising, went to the house of the second little pig with perverse, culinary intentions. Apparently this time just
one huff and puff wasn't enough for the big bad wolf, and he had to try
harder, although the result was the same: pig number two went from being
happy to being roasted, just like what had happened to his colleague in the
straw house. The third pig had been well alerted by the authorities about the
danger the wolf posed to pigs and to little girls walking through the woods
with baskets filled with goodies for their grandmothers. It is true that the
other two pigs had also been notified – the municipal edict was very clear

about it – but the third little pig stood out for his intelligence, prudence and spirit for survival. So he took the municipal warnings very seriously, and did so with effort and sacrifice, and also with hope, because he was aware that he was doing something that was going to benefit him most of all. So he built a nice, solid house out of bricks, with a proper security system, satellite dish and running water. When the wolf, who had become hungry again, tried to blow down the door, the house resisted. And it held up just fine against the wolf's other conscientious attacks. He tried everything: huffing and puffing harder, pounding on the door with a mallet, and pretending to be an encyclopedia salesman. Everything he did was in vane. Because of the third pig's prudence and intelligence, he was never eaten by the wolf and lived happily ever after with an attractive sow. He had seven beautiful little pigs and grew old peacefully until he died of a stroke at the age of 87.

We can tell a similar tale about three little pigs who had bipolar disorder. The first one simply did not believe what his veterinarian told him and thought that bipolar disorder was an illness that had been made up by psychiatrists or was a fairy tale, so he never changed the way he behaved: he'd jump around at all hours of the night, consume toxic substances whenever he had a chance, wouldn't pay attention to his friends when they warned him he was being too jittery and, of course, didn't take any of the medications he'd been told to take. The result of his attitude toward his disorder was that he suffered from constant relapses, even several a years, and this resulted in numerous stays at the hospital. He lost his job, his friends no longer paid attention to him because sometimes he was really very irritable and other times he'd say strange things about maybe really being a chicken and not a pig, and he was even arrested one time for disorderly conduct when he was trying to lay an egg in the town's hen house. The second little pig in the story agreed to take the medication his psychiatrist suggested, even more so at his family's insistence, and he considered the possibility that he really did have bipolar disorder. The mistake he made was in thinking that medication alone would help keep his mood stable, and so he took his medication the right way. However, he led an unorganized life, going against his psychologist's orders: he got little sleep, sometimes because he was studying and sometimes because he was out dancing salsa, he drank enough alcohol to alter his mood and tended to smoke joints, even though they are hard to roll when you have hooves instead of fingers.

All of this led him to suffer several relapses, even though he was taking his medication correctly. The third pig joined a psychoeducation group for little bipolar pigs. This activity, in addition to reasonable behavior and being highly motivated not to relapse (he knew he enjoyed life a lot more during periods of euthymia), led him to take all the necessary precautions to avoid the dreaded relapses: he took his medication and paid attention to his doctor's orders and those of his psychologist. He went out some nights, but he tried to get enough sleep. He never took any kind of toxic substances. He always paid attention to his wife's comments when he was being more nervous than usual, and he even learned to identify the signs of relapse in time. He was aware that this attitude involved scarifies, but since he was a smart little pig, he understood that it was worthwhile to live a moderate life in exchange for something so important as his happiness and personal stability. Out of all of the little pigs in this story, he was the wisest pig of all, and there are some who say that some pigs are smarter than people."

- Patients are generally relieved when they learn the high prevalence rate of bipolar disorders, because to some extent they stop feeling like "weirdoes." To reinforce this idea, we comment that although the official prevalence rate of the disorder is between 1% and 2%, more recent studies offer data that the prevalence rate is near 4% and studies on the bipolar spectrum show that the prevalence rate in the general population is above 10%.
- Some ideas that are usually uncomfortable for our patients are chronicity, recurrence, and "incurability." This forces us to be particularly prudent, although clear, when using these terms. As for chronicity, we can use the example of other chronic medical diseases that, when controlled the right way, allow a person to have a good quality of life (i.e. diabetes), and try to separate this idea from degenerative diseases, because many of our patients associate both terms. As for recurrence, the example of *The Three Little Pigs* can convey to our patients the idea that, although the disorder tends to come back periodically, whether or not they relapse often depends on their attitude toward the disorder (pharmacological adherence, following sleep guidelines, early detection of episodes), although we should avoid creating false expectations, since we professionals all know that strict adherence with pharmacological and behavioral guidelines does not guarantee long-term stability 100%. In any event, we have to make it clear to our patients that

although it is true that they may relapse even if they do everything right, relapses will always be less frequent, last less time and be less intense than if they had a different outlook. The term "incurability" is of particular concern to patients, because many of them deduce that they are always going to be depressed or manic. So we should clarify that the disorder is not curable in the sense that it cannot be "erased from the map," but that it can be kept in check – or "dormant," as some of our patients like to say – for long periods of time.

## Patient material

Bipolar disorder results from a change in the mechanisms that regulate mood. It appears that the limbic system is the area in the brain in charge of acting as an authentic "mood-o-meter," similar to the thermostat you have in your house: it keeps the temperature steady and activates the structures needed to maintain equilibrium. In the case of the thermostat, when it detects a temperature higher than the one it has been set at, it activates the air-conditioning unit and, in turn, it activates the heater if the temperature is excessively low. A person's mood tends to be regular and dependent on their environment. When people are suffering from bipolar disorders, that is when their "mood-o-meter" is not working properly; their mood becomes unstable, variable, and independent from their environment.

Bipolar disorder is an *hereditary disorder*, but this does not mean that there is a 100% probability that the child of a person who has bipolar disorder will also have it. In fact, the odds of the child not having the disorder are higher than those of having it, although logically the probability of someone having the disorder is higher than for the child of a person who does not have the disorder. On the other hand, the odds would also vary depending on the degree of family relationship.

There are several physiological mechanisms involved in bipolar disorders, most of them at the neurotransmitter level. Neurotransmitters are the substances in charge of carrying information in the brain. There is empirical evidence that some neurotransmitters (dopamine, serotonin, noradrenalin, acetylcholine) work abnormally in bipolar disorders. There are also abnormalities in hormonal functioning, most of all in the thyroid hormone. We can currently say without a doubt that *bipolar disorder has a biological base and is transmitted genetically*. Theories that said that different psychological or social factors (childhood trauma, poor family relationships, personality factors) caused bipolar disorder are no longer valid. We now know that all these factors can bring on the disorder or make it worse, but never cause it.

*Bipolar disorder is chronic and recurrent*: This means that it is with you in your entire life, although it is not as severe at all stages in your life, and that the episodes tend to repeat themselves.

Nearly 4% of the population suffers from some kind of bipolar disorder. Although many people believe otherwise, the truth is that bipolar disorder is a disorder that has existed throughout history, meaning that it is as old as human kind itself. The prevalence rates of this disorder are very similar in all countries, which demonstrates that it is a universal disorder, in no way linked to cultural or social circumstances.

Fortunately, *today we have very effective treatments* to keep bipolar disorders in check, so that many people who would have in the past spent a large part of their time on the fringes of society or institutionalized can now lead normal lives (in other words, they are not slaves to their disorder). Many bipolar patients lead entirely well-adjusted social, family and sentimental lives and hold jobs just as well as anyone who is not bipolar. In fact, the list of people affected by bipolar disorder who now hold prominent places in history is endless: political leaders like Churchill, painters like Van Gogh, Gauguin or Pollock, brilliant composers like Schumann or Tchaikovsky, jazz musicians as Charles Mingus, renowned writers like Virginia Wolf, Hemingway, Charles Baudelaire, Herman Hesse or Edgar Allan Poe, etc.

We must start thinking that having a bipolar disorder does not have to be any more or less serious than having other chronic diseases like asthma or diabetes, and that *for the most part the disorder can be kept in check through proper medication and by strictly following behavioral guidelines.*

---

### Assignment 1

In your opinion, what is the cause of your disorder? What other factors do you think can trigger your relapses?

# Session 3

# Etiological and triggering factors

## Goal

The basic goal of Session 3 is to have patients learn about the biological nature of their disorder and, above all, to learn to distinguish between the "causal" concept of the disorder, which we always emphasize as biological- and the "triggering" concept, which can be either biological or environmental. This distinction plays a basic role in the way many patients handle the feelings of guilt they have about their disorder, given that they believe they are suffering from bipolar disorder because of some factor they are responsible for and that acted as a trigger; for example, the consumption of toxic substances, stress, or interrupted sleep.

Although Session 3 is considered as part of Unit 1 (Awareness of the Disorder), it also covers aspects relative to Unit 3 (Avoiding Substance Abuse, see p. 147). Working on the topic of attributions is particularly relevant in patients whose feelings can fluctuate between feeling guilty and feeling no responsibility at all. Making a special emphasis on the biological nature of the disorder can have an unwanted effect. It can lead patients to blame all of their behavior on their disorder and adopt an attitude ranging from victimism, learned helplessness, or "passiveness," depending on each patient's personality.

## Procedure

- Although we are going to begin the session, like we always do, with an informal discussion and review questions that may have come up regarding the material and contents of Session 2, we should be cautious not to let the discussion carry on too long or fall into the trap of answering endless general questions about the disorder that patients might ask.
- After that, we should follow by presenting the topic of the day. In Session 3, it would be useful to have some kind of an illustrative slide or drawing

where patients can see a representation of the human brain and where the limbic system is clearly marked, because this is going to be very important in our discussion about the causes of bipolar disorder. If no resource of this kind is available, you can draw a sketch of the limbic system yourself on the blackboard (good luck with it, by the way).

- We will also be using the blackboard to clearly separate the causes and triggers into two columns. We can begin the session by asking our patients what they think the causes of their disorder are, and by doing so go over the take-home exercise we suggested they do last week. It is common for patients to mention a trigger instead of a cause, for them to say, for example, "I took cortisone and I felt bad" or "my wife left me and I got depressed." We will take that opportunity to make the distinction between both concepts.
- Playing a game to invert causes and effects is normally a very useful activity in this session.
- We can propose that the group debate blame vs. responsibility, by contrasting how thoughts of blame are useless and unproductive, and how useful, on the other hand, feelings of responsibility are.
- We will then go around the room for questions and, once this is done, we will end the session, but not before handing out the material and take-home assignment.

## Useful tips

- As always, it is very important that we do not take anything for granted. When we talk about genes, we should explain what we mean in very simple terms. Although some of the members of the group might have a scientific background, for example, we should not forget to move forward at a pace that is right for everyone.
- Although uncommon, we might get a reaction from some of our patients when they find out their illness is hereditary. They might blame their parents and express this feeling with phrases like "they could have thought twice about having me," "they could have given me some other inheritance, a house or something," which are phrases usually said jokingly. But sometimes you might hear more serious comments like "they've done me a huge injustice, and I'm not going to forgive them for it." The therapist must be aware of that possibility and be able to redirect the subject matter

if he detects a hostile reaction, by simply explaining that parents cannot decide what diseases their children are going to inherit, just like it is not up to them whether their children are going to inherit their father's eyes, their mother's cheeks, or the way their grandfather walks.

- It is important to make it clear that episodes can appear without there being any trigger (saying otherwise would not be the truth), and we should try to prevent patients from crossing the thin line separating being able to correctly identify a trigger and blaming themself for it. As we will see later on, the therapist must try to make the patient learn to accept responsibility and stop blaming themself. Even though we are going to have to work on the cognitions of blame if they appear, from a psychoeducation standpoint there is little we can do about blame – although providing information is usually quite powerful – but, on the other hand, co-responsibility is one of the engines of therapeutic alliance. Even though we are going to schematically, but thoroughly explain the phenomenon of kindling whereby the disorder tends to become separate from environmental triggering factors, we should especially stress what a patient can do for themself. And this is perhaps one of the most winding and troubled parts of the psychoeducation journey: an excessively biological view of the disorder can cause patients to feel that they cannot do anything except take medications and can even install in them a certain degree of victimism or a self-justifying attitude. Against what we have just said, we also cannot give our patients too much of an environmentalist view of the disorder, first of all because it is false, and also because it can lead somewhat easily to poor treatment adherence and to becoming confused about the diagnosis and blame.
- Prevalence data should be updated constantly, and comments about the prevalence of the different forms of the bipolar spectrum should be included. The data that places the prevalence of bipolar disorder near 4% of the general population come from the most recent studies (Hirschfeld et al., 2003), but we have been changing the prevalence rate figures in the different groups over the last 10 years.

## Patient material

We now know that genetics play a fundamental role in bipolar disorders. In fact, we can safely say that the cause of this disorder is genetic; that is to say, it is marked by the genes. This notion can be strange to us, in principle, because the disorder might not manifest itself until adulthood or because it might occur when no similar case is known in the affected person's family. The fact of the matter is that in order for certain illnesses with a hereditary component to manifest themselves, certain environmental factors need to occur that are just as important or more important than genetics is, and that is why the disorder does not manifest itself from birth. On the other hand, family background can also be very remote and, because of this, the affected person may not be aware of it. This is particularly common in psychiatric disorders because they have been so misunderstood for so many years, on the one hand, and because of the social taboo they have meant, which has been why a lot of families try to *hide* or make excuses for ill family members instead of trying to get them treatment. Mutations (spontaneous changes in genes) explain how hereditary illnesses can appear in individuals who have no family history of the disorder.

Generally speaking, although there are exceptions, the disorder begins to become just barely noticeable during adolescence (a stage that in and of itself causes emotional instability) and reaches its peak in adulthood, when it manifests itself as a depressive or manic phase. In any event, a person is at the highest risk of having his or her first episode when he or she is under the age of 50.

*Oftentimes, the first episode is preceded by an environmentally stressful situation.* From that moment on, the disorder begins to separate itself from environmental and psychological circumstances, so that the biological mechanisms regulating mood appear to perpetually swing back and forth, and make the affected person lose the reference point for his or her normal mood.

*With every relapse, the affected person becomes more vulnerable* to stress, and this makes some patients have rapid cycling, which is the uninterrupted succession of depression and euphoria (people who have four or more episodes a year).

In summary, we have to keep in mind, on the one hand, the *genetic factors* that are responsible for a person being vulnerable to suffer from a particular disorder and, on the other hand, the *factors implied in stress response.* In the case of bipolar disorder, we should underscore the importance of the genetic component and the fact that the factors implied in stress response are responsible for the disorder appearing and for accelerating new episodes. Some possible triggers are the death of a close relative or job changes, although it is also true that relapses can occur without anything unpleasant or traumatic having occurred (job promotion, change of address, etc.).

Bipolar disorder is slightly more common in women than it is in men, but rapid cycling is much more frequent in female patients.

*Approximately 4 out of every 100 people will suffer a bipolar disorder in their lives.* This risk is higher in people with relatives who have this disorder. In men, it is more likely for the first episode to be manic, and in women, a major depressive episode is more likely.

---

**Assignment 2**

Have you ever been diagnosed with a hypomanic or manic episode? What do you remember about that time? Try to describe what your behavior was like, your thoughts and your emotions.

---

# Symptoms I: Mania and hypomania

## Goal

The goal of Session 4 is to have patients come into contact for the first time with what a manic or hypomanic episode is. We have grouped mania and hypomania into the same session because of their clinical similarities. Ideally, we should also have included mixed episodes here, because from a clinical standpoint and – most of all – a therapeutic and psycho-social impact standpoint, mixed phases resemble mania more than they do depression. Mixed episodes were included in Session 5 (see p. 85) due to time constraints and to the fact that it does not look sensible to try to explain mixed phases before the patient has heard about both mania and depression. The purpose of Session 4 is not to teach patients how to detect a manic or hypomanic episode in time, but rather it simply tries to show them what a hypomanic or manic episode is. To do this, it is important in this session that we go directly to explaining the possible symptoms, without getting sidetracked into talking about the signs of relapse.

## Procedure

- As always, we will begin the session informally and open the group up to questions about last session.
- After the warm-up period, we can start by asking how many of the people in the room know what the word "mania" means, because each language may have different meanings for this word which may cause patients to become a lot more confused than what many professionals suspect (we should compare, for instance the meaning of the word "manic" with "maniac"). You can bring this into the discussion: a patient who suffers from mania is said to be manic, not a maniac. These distinctions can seem commonplace to us, but

they are not, and for many of our patients this will be decisive in order for them to better understand or accept their diagnosis.

- We can continue the session by asking how many in the room have suffered mania or hypomania. Before any questions are asked about the disorder that the patients, in our opinion, might consider to be indiscreet, it is important that we make it clear that "you do not have to answer and you will not be better or worse patients if you do answer." This and another appraisal of a similar nature will not make our patients feel that a part of their intimacy that some of them feel is embarrassing is being invaded. Patients who have done the take-home assignment can read a paragraph from the assignment if they want to.
- Before we begin our explanation about mania and hypomania, we will suggest going around the room to talk about the symptoms the patients have (Table 5), and we will write them all down on the blackboard. If we notice that everyone in the group is participating fully, we will allow the process to be spontaneous (meaning that participants will shout out a symptom when its comes to their mind, in no particular order). On the other hand, if we notice that the group is unevenly distributed and there are a few patients speaking up while the rest of the group is silent, which is usually what happens, we will direct the group to take turns, starting with the participant to our left and going around the circle clockwise. All patients should give a symptom of mania or hypomania, and we will go around the room as many times as necessary until all symptoms have been virtually exhausted. If a patient makes a mistake and gives a symptom of depression, we will immediately correct him or her, or we could let the group act as the correction team.
- We will then go on to present the material for the session.
- We will open a discussion and question period.
- After we have handed out the material and take-home assignment, we will close the session.

## Useful tips

- During the session we should openly stress the pathological nature of both mania and hypomania, since many of our patients see hypomania as "a blessing" or "a gift." In these instances, it would be useful for us to remind them that: (a) during hypomania people usually make the wrong decisions,

**Table 5.** Most frequent symptoms of mania and percentage of bipolar patients presenting them

| Symptoms | Bipolar patients presenting it (%) |
| --- | --- |
| Increased activity | 100 |
| Elevated "high" mood | 90 |
| Decreased need for sleep | 90 |
| Loquacity | 85 |
| Racing thoughts | 80 |
| Increased self-esteem | 75 |
| Being easily distracted | 65 |
| Increased sex drive | 60 |
| Irritability | 45 |
| Psychotic symptoms | 40 |
| Alcohol abuse | 35 |

(b) not all of the symptoms of hypomania are pleasant (i.e. many patients suffer while they are in a hypomanic phase because they are oversensitive, have rapid thoughts, or are restless, and (c) hypomania almost always leads to another immediate episode that involves greater suffering (mania, mixed phases, depression).

- We always recommend differentiating between hypomania and non-pathological happiness. A good exercise is to have patients give an example of each of these states. As the therapist, you can comment on the following differences (modified from Akiskal, 1997):
  - Hypomania does not have an apparent cause and its intensity is not disproportional to that cause. In turn, we are usually able to identify the reason why we feel happy.
  - Hypomania is labile: the person who has it is irritable and hostile when he or she is contradicted, something that does not happen in a person who is simply happy.
  - The intensity of the hypomania can lead a patient to try to get away from it by self-medicating or using sedatives or alcohol.
  - Hypomania tends to reduce a person's judgment; happiness does not.
  - Hypomania is typically preceded or followed by inhibited depression.
  - Hypomania is recurrent; unfortunately, happiness is not.

- When we write down the list of symptoms on the blackboard, we will more or less use the wording patients have provided in addition to the medical term to define the symptom (i.e. hearing voices/auditive hallucinations, "fast ideas"/racing thoughts, etc.). This is important because, on the one hand, we should use a language that closely matches what the patients are using and, on the other hand, we would like to have our patients have an understanding of the medical language. A lot of patients become distressed when they come across terms that they do not understand whenever they ask their psychiatrist for a writing report on their condition.

- We should emphasize that not all symptoms have to be present for there to be a hypomanic or manic episode. Furthermore, most often only some of them are present. By making this clear, we can avoid some of the excuses our patients may offer, which are often a reaction to the onset of a new episode when they say "I agree. I'm sleeping less than I should and I'm a little more irritable and anxious, but I'm not spending money," which shows that they are using their knowledge about their disorder to reinforce their denial.

- We should be especially careful when we explain the symptoms of psychosis, because these involve a significant part of the social stigma. Generally speaking, it is very positive to explain that we must not single out the psychotic symptoms of bipolar disorder any more than we do any other symptom in any other disorder. Given the fact that more or less half of our patients have suffered psychotic symptoms, it would be appropriate for us to be aware of and prevent our explanations about it from causing patients who have not had psychotic symptoms to react improperly to the rest of the group; for example, by considering them to be the most serious patients, to laugh at them or to pull away from them. We have all seen this kind of reaction in our psychoeducation groups, and they should be quickly and bluntly terminated and corrected by the therapist.

- Psychotic symptoms bring about diagnostic doubts not just among our patients, but also among some professionals. It would be appropriate for us to explain the differences between bipolar disorder and other psychotic disorders, for example schizophrenia, and to try to do so without reinforcing the stigma associated with schizophrenia, which means that you will have to stay away from such worn-out phrases like "schizophrenia is a much more serious disorder because it implies impairment," because doing this would only result in the opposite of what we want to achieve, which is to prevent fear and to do away with the stigma about mental disorder. An explanation that is usually convincing to our patients is that bipolar disorder and schizophrenia are two different disorders that share certain kinds of symptoms – psychotic symptoms – just like the flu and an infection might also share symptoms like a fever and continue to be two clearly separate illnesses.

• Another particularly delicate topic is the barrier that exists between psychotic symptoms and religious beliefs, which is something that a lot of the patients ask about. The questions that are usually asked have to do with whether appearances of the Virgin Mary or another type of divine representation on earth are really hallucinations, or to what extent are they a "direct line" to God or the sudden illuminations some of our patients experience during their manic phases. When answering these question, we should be especially careful not to offend believers. If the "illumination" is isolated and there is no other kind of accompanying symptom (something that is so infrequent we have yet to see it), the issue surely warrants more theological attention than psychiatric attention. What often happens is that mystic or religious exaltation presents itself in the context of a manic episode and it is nothing more than one of its symptoms, so that it goes away when the mania is treated. To explain this point easily and amicably, we usually joke about it and say that "we don't have a problem with you talking to God through prayer, but we would be worried if you actually heard Him answer you."

## Patient material

As we have already said, bipolar disorder is an alternation of depressive episodes, asymptomatic phases and episodes of euphoria. Today we are going to deal with the latter, which go by the name mania or hypomania, depending on their intensity.

Mania is an abnormal, persistently high or irritable state of mood. It is characterized by the following symptoms: increased *self-esteem*, decreased need to sleep, verbosity, *rapid* thinking, being easily distracted, psychomotor *agitation*, underestimating the risk and implication of pleasant activities that can have potentially serious consequences. Not all of these symptoms have to be present, in that there can be depression without sadness, manias in which *irritability* and anger overshadow happiness.

Nevertheless, we have to recognize that one of the most classic symptoms of manic episodes is increased self-esteem, which can run from self-confidence lacking self-critique to an obvious grandiose notion that attains delirious proportions. For example, people who are affected by this disorder can offer tips about things they know nothing about, they could write novels, compose a symphony or look to publish an invention that has no practical use. *Delirious grandiose notions* are common (i.e. having a special relationship with God or with a political, religious, or entertainment figure, having some kind of special power or virtue, etc.).

There always tends to be a *decreased need for sleep*: the person who is affected usually wakes up several hours earlier than usual feeling full of energy. When the sleep disorder is serious, the patient can go several days without sleep without feeling tired.

*Language* is typically *verbose, fast and hard to interrupt, and the person usually talks loudly*. What the person talks about is usually characterized by the addition of jokes, puns and somewhat funny remarks. The person can be theatrical, with dramatic mannerisms and songs. If the mood is predominantly irritable, the discourse will be riddled with complaints or hostile comments.

Another classic symptom is increased *thinking speed*, which some patients have defined as "watching two or three TV programs at once." Thoughts tend to come about faster than they can be put into words or even understood, and thought might be completely disorganized.

In some patients, increased sexual desire is common. This characteristic, along with not assessing the negative consequences of their behavior, leads many people to break their sentimental relationships during manic episodes and to have numerous sexual relationships, promiscuity and other sexual behavior uncommon for them.

Oftentimes, symptoms like expansivity, optimism without any reason, grandiose, and poor judgment lead to careless engagement in pleasant activities like unlimited shopping, fearful behavior, and unreasonable economic investments (accumulating a lot of unnecessary things: expensive antiques, 20 pairs of shoes, etc.).

Subjects suffering a manic episode *do not recognize that they are ill* and they might resist attempts at treatment. They frequently justify or rationalize their behavior, they travel impulsively to other cities, change the way they dress, their makeup or their personal appearance to a flashier or sexually suggestive style that may be inappropriate. They also behave strangely, offering advice about things they do not know anything about or giving away money. All of this can be accompanied by pathological gambling, antisocial behavior, and toxic substance abuse. Ethical considerations are oftentimes forgotten, and the people seem unaware of the feelings of others.

Irritability or inability to accept opinions and stances contrary to their own are not uncommon, and this can lead to verbal or physical abuse against objects (breaking things) or people. In spite of this and despite the alarming connotation that the press gives to the word "manic," we should indicate that significant aggression is uncommon during the manic phase. Contrary to popular belief, mania is not usually dangerous or violent.

During manic phases, psychotic symptoms tend to appear. There are two kinds: hallucinations (perception without an object to motivate it, that is seeing things or people, hearing voices, etc.) and delirium (more or less absurd or unfounded beliefs that go against all reason, that is, believing that you are fluent in a language you have never studied, believing you are being pursued by the KGB, or that the FC Barcelona Soccer Team has offered you a multi-million dollar contract to be their next forward).

---

### Assignment 3

Have you ever been diagnosed with a depressive or mixed episode? What do you remember about that time? Try to describe how you behaved and the thoughts and emotions you had.

---

# Session 5

# Symptoms II: Depression and mixed episodes

## Goal

The goal of Session 5 is to convey to our patients the idea that depression is a medical illness, moving away from pejorative social considerations or popular meanings associated with the term that lead one to believe that depression is caused by a person's surroundings and that it can be resolved by the person him or herself, without needing to consult a professional or receive treatment. Therefore, we will impart just the opposite message: depression is an illness or – the point in case – part of an illness that has clearly defined biological causes and generally requires pharmacological treatment. We will again insist on the need to differentiate normal emotions from pathological ones.

## Procedure

- To begin the session, after we have greeted group members, we go around the room and have patients ask questions about the last session.
- It is a good idea to start the session by reading some news articles (from recent newspapers or magazines) that improperly use the word "depression," something that unfortunately is not uncommon. There are plenty of headlines in the press like "Manchester United Goes Through November Depression: Five Defeats Straight" or "Katia, Very Depressed After Being Eliminated From *Big Brother*." We will invite the patients to give their opinion about the use of the unspecialized press makes of psychiatric terms, particularly the word "depression." This will give us a way to introduce the medical concept of depression, in terms that it is a biological illness and does not necessarily require triggering factors for it to appear.

- Even though we already discussed the causes and triggers of bipolar disorder in a previous session (see Session 3, p. 73), it would be a good idea to review them when we talk about depression, because most patients tend to make psychogenic attributions to their depressions, which is something that does not happen as often with manic episodes. Many bipolar patients believe that they suffer from depression solely and exclusively as a result of problems they are having with their partners or problems at work. It would be a good idea for us to give patients a way of looking at this in another way: maybe the patient did not become depressed because he lost his job or because his wife left him, but he lost his job and his wife because he was depressed.

- Another fundamental issue is for patients to learn not to necessarily identify depression with extreme sadness. Many bipolar patients do not see themselves in the classic popularized descriptions that characterize depression as a period of hopelessness and despair, which are aspects that are usually more typical of unipolar depression. On the other hand, we know that bipolar depression is characterized by alterations that are more behavioral (apathy, anergy, hypersomnia) than cognitive. So we should alert our patients about the existence of "sadless depression," because if patients use depressive sadness as a standard rule, they frequently get help too late when they are depressed. Sadness can be or is usually present, but it is not a *sine qua non* condition for there to be a depressive episode.

- We can continue the session by asking how many in the room have suffered depression, telling the members of the group, as we always do, that answering the question is completely optional. We can have volunteers present the assignments they did at home. We might be surprised to see that some of our bipolar patients say that they have never been depressed, even though we have probably documented episodes of depression in their case histories. They say this either because "they forget" about certain episodes or because, in the case of more "behavioral" depressions, patients associate them with some kind of physical ailment.

- After that, we can suggest going around the room and ask patients to list the symptoms of depression (Table 6), and we will write down all the ones they mention on the blackboard. Once again, we will use the expressions the patients give as well as the clinical terms they are referring to.

**Table 6.** Most frequent symptoms of depression and percentage of bipolar patients presenting them

| Symptoms | Bipolar patients presenting it (%) |
| --- | --- |
| Sadness | 86 |
| Loss of energy | 86 |
| Difficulty concentrating | 79 |
| Negative cognitions | 64 |
| Decreased sleep | 57 |
| Loss of interest | 57 |
| Weight loss | 43 |
| Weeping | 43 |
| Loss of appetite | 36 |
| Somatic symptoms | 36 |
| Irritability | 29 |

- The next step after we have completed the list of symptoms is to explain in detail what each symptom consists of, placing special emphasis on differentiating them from non-pathological mood variations. So, for example, if we are talking about anhedonia, we can comment that, obviously, there will be days when we will enjoy our pleasant activities less without being depressed, but that anhedonia refers to a person's inability to enjoy any activity and that, in any event, it is easier to evaluate it if it is accompanied by other symptoms. As for fatigue, we should comment that a depressed person's fatigue is not associated with any effort, unlike the normal fatigue that occurs after a person has been physically active. Sadness is also a normal emotion that can be a symptom of depression, and when this happens, it is generally disproportional to any stimulus and does not change or get better. The only symptom that is not a continuation of normality is suicidal ideation and, therefore, we can consider that it alone is indicative of a depressive episode.
- At the end of the session, we will open it for discussion. A lot of patients want to explain how they have felt when they were depressed, because for the first time in their lives they feel they are in the right place: they are with people like them who have suffered *to their very cores* the same thing that

the rest of them have gone through, which is something that does not take place when they are with their therapist.

## Useful tips

- We can spend some time having patients comment about the repercussions depressive episodes have had on their family, social, and job-related lives, as well as how they have suffered by being considered lazy, when in reality, they are sick, and they can share some of their intimate experiences associated with depression. All this is not one of the objectives of the group *per se*. A patient who has experienced depression usually says to the psychiatrist something like "you could never understand me completely because you have never been depressed like me." So then now we can offer patients a chance to talk about their depression with people who have suffered from it just like them. This gives many bipolar patients a great sense of relief and they stop feeling so alone, and they are also able to conceptualize depression as part of the disorder and recognize that the symptoms and experiences they have had are shared by most of the people in the group. How many of our patients have told us during a one-on-one visit something like "You can't help me because you don't know what this is like"? Obviously, any minimally trained clinician has enough resources available to combat this argument, but it does not stop being true that patients feel like that and that is what they say. The feeling that the clinician is never going to be able to truly understand how a patient feels can lead a depressed patient to fall into nihilistic attitudes regarding the success of a particular treatment, regardless of whether the treatment consists mainly in pharmacotherapy or psychotherapy, and could even lead the patient to feel that he has never been so sick and he is never going to recover. Having contact with other patients is useful in preventing this nihilism.
- Information about the pathological nature of depression is usually very guilt releasing, because patients have often been accused of being "weak" or "lazy" by the people around them while they were depressed. So, logically there is a certain anger toward the people who say such things that goes along with the exoneration. To redirect this anger, we can remind our patients that just as they were unaware of what depression represented until they had it, their family members and friends have no reason to be experts on or even familiar with this issue.

- Once we have commented on the sleeping problems that are usually associated with depression, we can introduce the topic about the therapeutic use of sleep. So, trying to get 9 h of sleep a night can be very useful to overcome a depressive episode. In any event, this topic will come up again in future sessions (see p. 180).
- An issue that should be discussed openly is suicide. In fact, when the group is more advanced, we can usually give them specific information about this issue, which we always treat as one more symptom of depression, divesting it of any philosophical or literary device. We have to make it clear to our patients that suicide is not a right, but rather a complication of the disorder, and prevent them from associating such vastly different issues like suicide and euthanasia, which some patients tend to bring up. Although it is not the primary objective, our experience has shown us that the group is usually able to integrate and contrast suicidal ideation. In fact, we have found that none of the more than 200 patients who as of now have received psychoeducation or unstructured intervention has committed suicide. That is to say, it is not that the concepts presented in the group *per se* have anti-suicidal properties, but weekly meetings of patients who have similar needs with a professional do appear to have an impact on this aspect.

## Patient material

The essential characteristic of a depressive episode is that it involves a period of at least 2 weeks during which there is a state of depressed mood or a *loss of interest or pleasure* for almost all activities. To consider that a person is suffering from depression – and not simply that he is sad or worried about negative events – there should also be present, in addition to *sadness or irritability*, another four symptoms from a list, which includes *changes in appetite* or weight, changes in sleep pattern (generally oversleeping, but also insomnia sometimes), slowing of movements, *fatigue*, loss of usual interests, *lack of energy, feelings of inferiority or guilt*, difficulty thinking, concentrating or taking decisions, and thoughts of death or ideas of suicide (Table 7).

Frequently, depressed people describe their mood as sad, hopeless, having the blues, like being "in a well." In spite of this, for bipolar depression it is also usual for the sadness not to be the dominant emotion and that in its place there is a sensation of inhibition, *emotional emptiness*, indifference, or passiveness.

**Table 7.** Symptoms and characteristics of the depressive phase

| Behavior | | Thoughts | | Emotions/sensitivity | |
|---|---|---|---|---|---|
| Symptoms | Characteristics | Symptoms | Characteristics | Symptoms | Characteristics |
| Insomnia/Hypersomnia | Motor restlessness, plus (rarely) agitation, which decreases job or academic performance (inactivity), and even produces isolation and distancing oneself from society and family. In serious cases of depression, we can even find bed confinement, depressive stupor, or suicide attempts. There is generally an inability to feel or experience pleasure and satisfaction and loss of interest in things. | Slowness | Behaves more slowly and has negative content, a pessimistic outlook on the past, present and future, and feelings of not being appreciated and guilt. In severe cases there can be delirious ideas of being useless, guilt, mayhem or, for example, thoughts leading the patient to believe he deserves to be punished. Problems with memory, attention and concentration are also seen. | The blues | Sadness, which may be expressed as indifference apathy, dejection or, more rarely as anxiety/ irritability. In some cases there is a kind of "numbing" sensation. |
| Loss/increased appetite | | Lack of concentration | | Sadness | |
| Physical discomfort | | Memory problems | | Irritability | |
| Motor inhibition | | Decreased attention | | Feeling of emptiness | |
| Motor restlessness | | Psychic anxiety | | Emotional indifference | |
| Fatigue | | Suicide ideation | | | |
| Apathy | | Delirious ideas | | | |
| Sexual withdrawal | | Hallucinations | | | |
| Lack of energy | | Pessimism | | | |

*Anxiety* is also common. Other depressed people place a special emphasis on their physical complaints (widespread discomfort or pain without any medical cause). Some show a heightened state of irritability (i.e. persistent anger, tendency to respond by insulting others, or feelings of frustration about things that are not important). As we can see, bipolar depression can take on various forms and still be the same illness.

We almost always find a noticeable lack of interest and ability to enjoy life. When a person is depressed, he or she tends to be less interested in activities that were usually gratifying (hobbies, going to the movies, theater or going for a walk, getting together with family and friends, etc.). In most cases, there is also a significant decrease or complete disinterest in sexual desire, although this is reversible. In some cases, the patient losses his or her appetite and must take great pains to eat. In other instances, the person is hungrier and eats without any order, usually candy and chocolate. As a result, there is the possibility of weight loss as well as weight gain.

Sleep alterations are very common: oversleeping or *hypersomnia* and drowsiness during the day. Sometimes the patient wakes up during the night and has a lot of trouble falling back to sleep (sleep maintenance insomnia) or sleeping (inability to sleep).

Psychomotor changes include *restlessness* (inability to stay seated for long periods of time, general anxiety, nervous hand movements), but also *slowing down* (language, thinking and movements are slower and the tone of voice is softer).

*Lack of energy*, feeling tired and fatigue are very common. People feel fatigue persistently without having done any kind of physical exercise, so that any easy task requires a lot of effort. The efficiency with which they carry out their daily tasks and routines is greatly reduced, for example taking care of themselves or hygiene, which can become so exhausting to the patient that he or she stops doing it.

Feelings of being useless or guilt involve a negative, unrealistic evaluation of oneself or feelings of guilt, and worry about past mistakes, even if they were insignificant. This can lead to patients misinterpreting trivial events, which they wind up considering as proof of the many personal flaws they think they have. It is common for there to be an exaggerated feeling of responsibility for adversities.

*Thoughts about death or suicide* are very common (one out of every three bipolar patients attempt suicide once in their life) and, although we will be discussing it in detail in another session, we can put forth that suicidal ideas are always a symptom of an illness. Among the reasons that lead depressed patients to consider attempting suicide are a desire to give up in the face of what they believe to be an insurmountable obstacle or put an end to a painful emotional state that they perceive – mistakenly – is going to last forever and cannot be fixed.

Depressive episodes can be preceded by psycho-social stress factors like the death of a loved one or separation. These events can trigger the episode, but not cause it. In most cases, however, these episodes occur spontaneously, without any stress factor being present. For women, having a baby can act as a trigger, just like it can lead to a manic episode, and menstruation can also become a factor to take into account.

We understand *mixed phases* to be ones where depressive symptoms are mixed together (i.e. pessimism, ideas about death or incapacity) with manic symptoms (agitation, restlessness, rapid thought), generally largely overshadowed by irritability, anxiety, lability, and restlessness.

# Evolution and prognosis

## Goal

The objective of the sixth session is to focus on the chronic and recurring character of the bipolar disorder, further emphasize the difference between cause and trigger, and remind the patient of the cyclic character of the disorder based on the mood-chart technique, which the patient must master by the end of the session.

## Procedure

- Before each session, we will give all patients detailed explanatory documentation on how to make up the life chart and six or seven invented examples which we will use during the session. This documentation may be left on the chair for each patient or delivered to them when they enter the session.
- We will start the session, like always, inviting the patients to ask questions about the content of the previous session. Since Session 5 was about depression, it would not be surprising if its contents had worried certain patients and make them recall during the week the traumatic or unpleasant experiences of the depressive episodes. If we suspect that this might have happened, we will try to be open to completely changing the content of the sixth session and leaving it for the following week, focusing on working with the negative emotions generated in the previous meeting. Even though it is desirable to conduct the program as planned, we must remember that our ultimate objective is not to transmit knowledge but to prevent relapses, and for this purpose it may be very useful to dedicate more than one session to particularly delicate topics such as the experience of depression.
- We will tell the patients that "today we will do something different, we will learn to represent our disorder graphically." This point is usually extremely interesting to them.

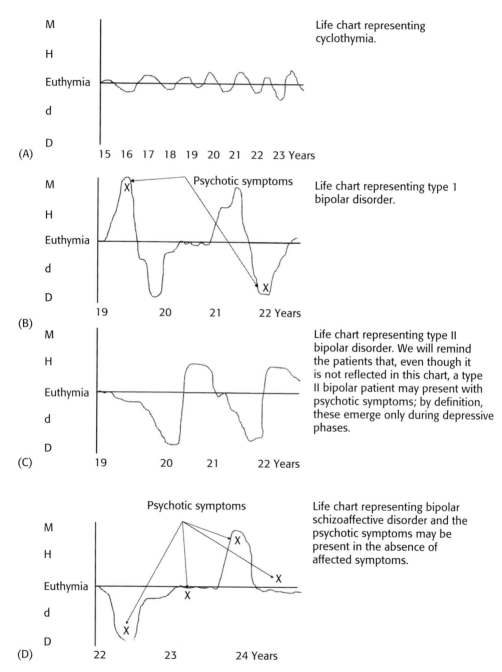

Life chart representing cyclothymia.

Life chart representing type 1 bipolar disorder.

Life chart representing type II bipolar disorder. We will remind the patients that, even though it is not reflected in this chart, a type II bipolar patient may present with psychotic symptoms; by definition, these emerge only during depressive phases.

Life chart representing bipolar schizoaffective disorder and the psychotic symptoms may be present in the absence of affected symptoms.

Figure 1    Life charts exemplifying the four types of bipolar disorders (A–D) (d: mild depression; D: severe depression; H: hypomania; M: mania).

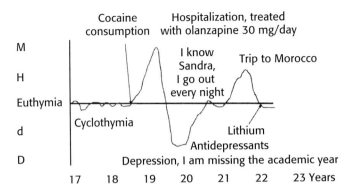

Figure 2    Life chart in which the patient noted the triggers, certain key treatments and facts (d: mild depression; D: severe depression; H: hypomania; M: mania).

- Using the blackboard we will explain to the members of the group how a life chart is done (see p. 101).
- To start giving examples of application of this technique, we will first explain the four types of bipolar disorders (type I, II, cyclothymia, and bipolar schizoaffective disorder), marking clearly the differences between them and representing them graphically (Figure 1A–D).
- Next, we will give ourselves an example of life chart, which we will invent with the help of the members of the group. They will suggest the incidences (episodes, triggers, consequences, treatments) suffered by the virtual patient, which, in turn, may serve to check up to what point the patients have understood the contents of the previous sessions (Figure 2).
- Next, we will review the examples we enclosed with the documentation. The patients themselves are in charge of explaining what they see in the life charts we provided. It is interesting for these examples to include a wide range of cases. We propose the following:
  - *Example 1*: Young patient who has his first relapse is, generally manic, associated to substance consumption (alcohol and cocaine). When he starts the treatment without stopping the consumption of toxics he continues suffering relapses. Finally, the evolution stabilizes when he stops consuming toxics, even though occasionally he may suffer depression or hypomania.
  - *Example 2*: Patient who has been treated for several years as unipolar and received only antidepressants. This causes him rapid cycling even

though he only comes to the doctor when he is depressed. When the patient is prescribed mood stabilizers, his evolution stabilizes. He normally presents with one depressive episode at Christmas and is "joyful" every summer.

– *Example 3*: Patient with unequivocal evolution of type II bipolar disorder who presents with psychotic symptoms in his depressive phases and stabilizes after adequate treatment.

– *Example 4*: Young patient who has been hospitalized several times after interrupting the medication and presenting with manic episode and a depressive episode with a suicide attempt. After a long hospitalization, the patient understands the need to follow the treatment, even though he has already lost his job and some of his friends.

– *Example 5*: Patient with sudden onset of the disorder, hospitalized for psychotic mania. After receiving medical treatment, he stays euthymic for several years, even though occasionally he presents with hypomania after exams period in which he slept very little.

– *Example 6*: Patient in whom all relapses are associated to psycho-social triggers. After getting a boyfriend, she starts presenting with manic symptoms, and after her mother's death presents with hypomania. In addition, 2 months after pregnancy she has depressive symptoms.

• We can choose to use only three of these examples and leave another three for another session, since this exercise is greatly liked by our patients. In fact, they often use a virtual case to express their anxieties, and this usually takes a lot of time.

• Many of the questions included in the documentation of the sixth session would have already appeared during our explanations of the life charts. However, we will complete the information with a brief chart lasting about 20 min.

• We will ask the patients who want to make a life chart of their own case or of an invented case (thus we will open the door to the presentation of their own case in a camouflaged manner). Those who decide to prepare their own life chart may get help from past reports or prescriptions, and complete the information with that given by a trusted person.

• We must warn our patients that making their own life chart is an intense emotional work, which implies stirring-up things from the past, so that we ask them to abandon it immediately if they start feeling uncomfortable, and to give them an opportunity to complete it in an individual session with the therapist.

- After the round of questions, we deliver the patient material, the two homework assignments, and we end the session.

## Useful tips

- It is important for patients not to misinterpret the life chart as a reductionist attempt to summarize their lives. In reality we, as well as they, are representing graphically the course of a disorder from which they suffer, not their lives, which are obviously much more complex.
- When we explain the various subtypes of bipolar disorders, it is recommendable not to give the impression that one subtype is more severe than another – except perhaps for cyclothymia, which would be less severe, since in this case, certain patients may play the role of one who is "not so ill," often leading to poor adherence; at the same time others quickly adopt, in a defeatist manner, the role of "complex patient." In reality, the degree of complexity of a case depends on such variables as the response to drugs, comorbidity (both psychiatric as well as axis III disorders), substance abuse, personality disorders or adherence; in addition, it is not clear that type II bipolar disorder is an attenuated form of type I, because, even though it is true that the episodes are across the board less severe in type II, it is also true that they are generally more frequent and often it is more difficult to obtain remission *ad integrum*.
- We will use the examples of the virtual life charts for more than one session, so that we must recommend to the patients to bring the documentation in the following sessions.
- The virtual charts may be used to focus on certain points that need to be emphasized. Example 1 will serve to emphasize the association between the consumption of toxics and relapses, and the fact that avoiding the conception of toxics is as important a part of the treatment as the drugs themselves. Example 2 may be used to insist on the fact that hypomania is *also* part of bipolar disorder and that not treating it is a serious mistake, both if it is the

consequence of incorrect diagnosis or if it is due to the fact that the patient does not consider it a problem. We will also represent the topic of the seasonal pattern associated with the changes in sunlight – and not social aspects such as Christmas or summer. Example 3 can be useful to remind the patient that, no matter how complex a case may be from a transverse viewpoint, long-term stabilization can be achieved. On the contrary, with Case 4 we will stress the complications that may be associated with the disorder if the patient is negligent in his treatment. In Case 5, we will remark on the one hand that even though the beginning of the disorder may be quite spectacular, it does not necessarily mean that the evolution will always be slow. In addition, we will use it to insist on the importance of the regularity of sleep. In Case 6, we will insist on the role of the triggers, emphasizing once again its differences from the causes. It will also serve to introduce the concept of postpartum depression – and mania – which will explain to our patients stressing that birth giving may act as a biological trigger (due to sudden hormonal changes) rather than psychological (which is what most our patients believe).

- When we work with life charts, both virtual and otherwise, we may use them to stress again the difference between cause and triggers (see Session 3, p. 73) asking the patients whether such-or-such events "caused" such depression. We will expressly use the verb "cause" to distinguish it from "trigger," and we will hope that the patients realize that an event never causes a phase, but often triggers it.

## Patient material

Bipolar disorders set in earlier than unipolar disorders (depressions without episodes of euphoria). They usually emerge *for the first time before age 30* and it is very unusual for the first episode to take place after age 50. The first episode may be both manic and depressive or mixed. The duration of the episode varies, even though it is rather constant for each patient.

*Without treatment*, the natural evolution of an episode prolongs from a few weeks to several months, but with treatment it is possible to shorten its duration so that an improvement is noticed 2–3 weeks after the beginning of the treatment in the case of the depressive episodes and a few days later in the case of manic episodes. The possibility for an episode to begin is much lower if the person who suffers from the disorder takes the medication correctly. If it still starts, the episode will be much less severe, it will have less consequences and will last for a shorter period of time. Continuing the treatment means reducing the risk of suffering an immediate change toward an episode of the contrary sign, for example from mania to depression.

After the first episode (mania, depressive or mixed) years may pass without any symptom being felt by the patient (euthymic), but we must take into account that bipolar disorder is a *recurrent disorder* which means that many of those who suffer from it will present with future episodes. This must not frighten us, because the possibility of controlling the relapses is in our hands, and has the importance of *following the pharmacological treatment prescribed* without underestimating, at all, the relevance of *our participation in this process* to avoid the relapses (consequently, it is fundamental to have information about the disorder, since this way we achieve better control, if not on the disorder itself, at least on its effect).

Certain effects or consequences of the disorder consist of the fact that various aspects of the person's life, such as marriage children, friends, or work may be affected.

Even though most persons who suffers from bipolar disorder return to total normalcy in the periods between episodes, some (20–30%) continue showing affective liability or instability and interpersonal or work difficulties. Once again, we will insist on the fact that both correct pharmacological treatment and psychotherapy help are fundamental to minimize the sequelae.

The manic episodes usually start suddenly, with a rapidly increasing symptoms over a few days. Frequently, they appear after some type of psycho-social stress, lasting from a few weeks to several months and in general are shorter and end more abruptly than the depressive episodes. In many cases, a depressive episode immediately precedes or follows a manic episode, without an intermediate period of euthymia. But what most often happens is that, after a manic episode, the person enters a "low" period that may be confused with a depressive episode. This picture is characterized by apathy, lack of energy, reduced attention, concentration and/or memory, hypersomnia, increase in appetite, etc. This is a period in which a person is dysphoric, and this condition must be fought by increasing the level of activity and not spending too much time in bed, otherwise this stage lasts much longer. It is better not to immediately use antidepressants, since there is a risk of decompensating the patient again toward a manic phase. In this stage of dysphoria, the patient has a sensation of malaise and feelings of guilt for what he has done during the manic episode.

The mixed episodes may emerge after a manic episode or a depressive episode, lasting between a few weeks and several months, and lead to a period with few or no symptoms, or may evolve toward a depressive episode. The evolution of a mixed episode toward a manic episode is much less frequent.

Hypomanic episodes start suddenly, with a rapid increase in symptoms, in 1 or 2 days. They usually last between a few weeks and several months, but are shorter and have a more sudden end than the depressive episodes. Many times, a hypomanic episode may be preceded or followed by a depressive episode. Existing studies suggest that 5–15% of the persons with hypomania will end up with a manic episode.

There are indications that changes in sleep–wake rhythm, such as those during travel or sleep deprivation may precipitate or exacerbate manic, mixed or hypomanic episodes. On the other hand, if in an episode, psychotic symptoms appear, it is most probable that they will reappear in subsequent episodes.

Depressive episodes tend to develop over days or weeks, but usually an untreated episode lasts 6 months or more. Almost always there is a complete remission of the symptoms and the activity returns to normal.

*After each new relapse, the person affected becomes more vulnerable* or likely to suffer new decompensation, that is the more episodes he experiences the more probable it is that he will suffer subsequent relapses; in addition, the time interval between an episode and the next becomes shorter and the duration of the episode increases.

*Rapid cycling*, which consists of presenting with more than 4 episodes a year, affects 10–15% of bipolar patients in some stage of their lives. This is a stage in which the evolution of the disorder becomes worse, but this worsening is reversible. We now know that the efficacy of lithium in these cases is not so high, but there are alternatives, such as carbamazepine, valproic acid, lamotrigine, or oxcarbazepine, which are also mood stabilizers, or we can add to the treatment a typical maintenance antipsychotic such as olanzapine, for example. On the other hand, there are indications that hyperthyroidism (deficient functioning of the thyroid) may play a role in the predisposition to rapid cycling. This is the reason why preventive checkups are done. Antidepressants may also act as triggers of rapid cycling so that they must be avoided whenever there are no marked or severe depressive symptoms. In the case of a dysphoric state, it is necessary to try to take the adequate dose of mood stabilizer and take behavioral measures: not becoming isolated, going out and meeting with friends, fulfill study and/or work obligations, the sooner the better, sleep for a limited period of time but not during the day, etc.

It is calculated that three-quarters of the patients hospitalized for mania will in the end be rehospitalized for a new episode. The *relapse prevention* strategy consisting of complying with the treatment and better knowing the disorder will lead, in the event of relapse, to a lower intensity and therefore a reduction in the possibility for rehospitalization, which is rather disruptive in itself.

## Make your own life chart

We call life-charts the graphic representation of the various episodes experienced by bipolar patients. Mastering the technique for making the life chart is relatively simple and very useful, since it will allow them to appreciate with a certain perspective the evolution of their disorder, its triggers and whether, for example, there are times of the year when the probability of a relapse is higher (e.g. spring, Christmas, final exams, etc.).

To prepare one's life chart, it is necessary to take the following steps:

- Draw on paper a "T" with the longer part horizontally, representing time, and with a shorter bar vertically, representing your mood: mania (M), hypomania (m or H), euthymia (E), mild depression (d), and severe depression (D). As to the period of time, it would be recommendable for your life chart to cover a limited period of time as possible, which should be highly relevant for the patient. Before starting to fill it out with your data, the appearance of the chart must be similar to that in Figure 3.
- After you do this, start to presenting the episodes graphically according to their intensity and duration. An upward curve will indicate hypomania (if it reaches H) or mania (if it reaches M); in the same way, a downward curve will indicate mild depression (d) or more severe depression (D). The separation between the lines will indicate the duration.

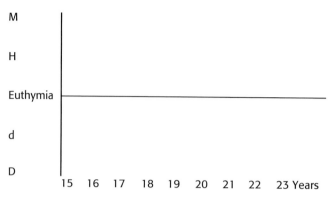

Figure 3   Axes presenting time and mood in a life chart.

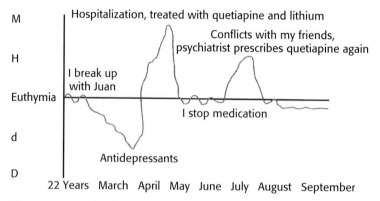

Figure 4   Example of notes to be made in the life chart, including possible triggers of an episode, consequences, treatment, etc. This chart will concretely correspond to the case of a young 22-year-old woman who apparently had the first depressive episode after she broke up with a boyfriend. It seems that, when treated with an antidepressant, she experienced a manic episode which required hospitalization. The patient was acceptably well during June and July, until she decided to stop taking the medication and started "going up" again, which took her to an important conflict with her friends. After consulting the psychiatrist, she resumed taking quetiapine and lithium and started improving slowly.

- For each episode, we should indicate whether there was a factor that may have acted as a trigger (splitting with partner, changing job, a trip, the death of a loved one, a new medication), what consequences it had (hospitalization, lost job) and what treatment was efficacious. Let us see a new example of these types of indications and their interpretation in Figure 4.

**Assignment 4**

Try to draw the chart of your disorder. If necessary, you can request the help of relatives or friends, or use reports in order to remember dates and events.

**Assignment 5**

Have you taken or are you taking any of the following drugs: lithium carbonate, sodium valproate, valpromide, lamotrigine, oxcarbazepine, carbamazepine, sodium levothyroxin? What do you think they are good for? Do they cause you any discomfort?

# Drug adherence

Improving treatment adherence must be one of the main objectives of any psychological intervention in bipolar disorders, since the problem of poor adherence is certainly the cornerstone of the poor evolution of many of our patients. The problem is severe if we consider that practically all bipolar patients seriously think at least once in their life of abandoning treatment, and it is not risky to affirm that more than half the patients stop taking the prescribed treatment without indication from their psychiatrists, even including during periods of euthymia. On the other hand, treatment withdrawal is the most common cause of relapse among bipolar patients and in fact, the risk of hospitalization is four times higher among the patients who do not duly comply with their maintenance treatment. Mortality, especially by suicide, is also higher in untreated patients. These considerations, along with the high rates of poor adherence recorded in bipolar populations, force us to make a great effort to improve our patients' adherence to treatment. This effort makes it appropriate for us to dedicate up to seven sessions to this topic in our program.

As we can see in Chart 1, when speaking of poor adherence we are not only referring to the patient who does not take his medication. Broadly, we can affirm that by poor adherence we understand that inability of the patient to follow some or all of the instructions given by his psychiatrist and psychologist, including drug prescription and the facilitation of health-promoting behavior or habits.

Several authors have described that the sudden interruption in taking lithium induces resistance to this drug in patients who initially respond to treatment, but this matter is still controversial. If this phenomenon of development of refractoriness is confirmed, we could speak of durable adverse consequences of treatment withdrawal, beyond the obvious increase in the risk of relapse and the number of hospitalizations.

**Chart 1. Types of poor treatment adherence**

1  *Absolute poor adherence.* This refers to the complete negligence of the patient in following the indications of the responsible therapist, or the refusal to visit the therapist. Probably, this is the least studied form of poor adherence, due to its very nature: the patient who absolutely does not take the medication rarely will duly comply with the scheduled visits with the psychiatrist, which makes it difficult to follow up and evaluate the real impact of these cases. If we only apply restrictively the criteria for absolute poor adherence to patients who reject treatment but continue coming to the appointments with their psychiatrist, we will obtain a percentage of above 10% (Colom et al., 2000) of bipolar patients who behave in this fashion, even when they are stable.

2  *Selective partial adherence.* Certain patients selectively reject a certain type of treatment but not another. When there is a problem of partial awareness of the disorder (this is the case of the patient who do not really believe in the chronic nature and the recurrent nature of their bipolar disorder), some patients propose to their psychiatrists to medicate them only with antidepressants during decompensations, instead of treating the disorder longitudinally. Other patients accept any type of treatment for the acute phase, including antipsychotics, but reject prophylactic treatment. At the other end, there will be those who accept to take lithium carbonate because they consider it something "natural" but refuse to take other drugs. The knowledge of the disorder and the fear of side effects are basic in understanding this type of behavior. Partially complying patients constitute a variable of confusion vs. the rates of non-responders in any study of the efficacy of a drug. The aspects related to adherence may explain the existing differences between the efficacy of lithium in controlled clinical studies and its efficacy in clinical practice or in naturalistic studies.

3  *Intermittent adherence.* Without any doubt, this discontinuous adherence is the rule among the patients who take lithium, rather than the exception (Maj, 1999). Many patients do not completely abandon the treatment but neither do they take it as prescribed. The patients with intermittent adherence allow themselves variable periods of "vacations from treatment"; during these periods, sometimes long, the patient partially or completely abandons all or some of the drugs prescribed to them, frequently offering such explicit reasons as "I would like to rest from the

medication." Some of these patients even learn to hide their non-adherence by taking high doses of mood stabilizers days before their serum levels are checked, with the risk it implies.

4 *Late adherence.* A very common pattern described by Goodwin and Jamison (1990): some patients show initial resistance to admitting the need to receive treatment and decides to start taking the medication prescribed after a few relapses. This would explain the relationship between the duration of the disorder and the adherence prescribed by certain authors (Colom et al., 2000).

5 *Late poor adherence.* After 2 or 3 years of good adherence, some patients start abandoning their mood stabilizers without apparent reason. This phenomenon has been described both with lithium (Jamison et al., 1979) and anticonvulsants (Adams and Scott, 2000).

6 *Abuse.* Contrary to common belief, poor adherence does not just mean taking less medication than prescribed. Taking more medication is also a rather common form of poor adherence among bipolar patients, especially if they also suffer from drug dependency (Weiss et al., 1998), or a personality disorder. The abuse of benzodiazepine is, obviously, very common (Woods et al., 1988), but it is only the tip of the iceberg: there are cases of abuse of antidepressants (Delisie, 1990), neuroleptics (Buckley, 1991) and even atypical antipsychotics (Vieta et al., 2001) and new anticonvulsants prescribed with mood-stabilizing aims (Colom et al., 2001). It is noteworthy that certain patients take more medication than prescribed because of their impatience to improve (Weiss et al., 1998).

7 *Behavioral poor adherence.* The term "poor adherence" does not only refer to pharmacological adhesion (which consists, among other things, in respecting intake times and correctly complying with the quantity indicated), but also includes aspects concerning the attitude and behavior of the patient during the visits: visits, giving the physician relevant and sufficient information about the case, obeying the clinician's instructions as to the regularity of sleep habits and other advisable behaviors that may facilitate euthymia, such as not consuming alcohol or other toxics. Certain patients correctly take the medications prescribed but fail to comply with behavioral indications, perhaps moved by an excessively biological idea of their disorder or simply by convenience; this also is closely related to a form of lack of awareness of the disorder, because the patient

is not willing to sacrifice part of their routine for a disorder he does not consider sufficiently severe, and it would explain why behavioral treatments focused on the disorder may improve the evolution of bipolar patients, including those who take the pharmacological treatment correctly, as we have reported (Colom et al., 2003a).

On the other hand, several authors have observed lower mortality rates among bipolar patients who correctly take the treatment prescribed, as compared to bipolar compliant patients, which is partially explained by the anti-suicide properties of lithium.

## Can we predict poor adherence?

Given the clinical relevance of the fact, we must make an effort to identify early the patient who is poorly adherent. As it happens with so many other clinical characteristics, the personal history of poor adherence probably constitutes the best predictor for the future. There are several factors associated to poor adherence in bipolar patients, as shown in Chart 1. Depending on the various studies, each factor will have more or less weight and, in this sense, the published data are still contradictory to date. On the one hand, the patients spontaneously present several reasons to abandon the treatments, among which we can stress the denial of the disorder, side effects, feeling uncomfortable for having to take a psychotropic drug, or missing the periods of euphoria. The attitudes toward the disorder and the health beliefs of each patient play a highly relevant role in the emergence of poor adherence: obviously, bipolar patients who firmly believe that they can control their mood by themselves will have a worse degree of adherence. On the other hand, adherence is better in patients who are informed of the potential negative consequences of their disorder and in those who are capable to identify the benefits of pharmacological treatment. Both complying patients and non-complying ones agree to consider fear of depression as the main reason to continue pharmacological treatment, above the fear of mania, even though there are exceptions naturally.

The social stigma, which unfortunately is associated with mental disorder, may make some patients abandon treatment because they are ashamed to take medication, they are worried because of misinformation, etc., and this makes the patient's environment a key part in the complex mechanism of therapeutic adherence. It seems that the opinion of those who surround the patient clearly; for instance, the patient's attitude toward the treatment. Family and interpersonal problems may constitute a path to poor adherence, especially in environments which by themselves offer little support.

Poor adherence has traditionally been associated with young patients, even though certain authors argue that age is relevant only in its extremes, in other words, adolescence and the elderly will be less compliant. Other demographic variables, such as being male and unmarried appear to be related in literature to poor adherence, even though this occurs with most diseases not only psychiatric ones. There is no agreement among researchers in this regard. Most of the studies do not find adherence differences according to gender, even though the most solid study of those made to-date about the reasons for poor adherence has found differences between genders concerning the abandonment of treatment. Women would be more likely to abandon treatment because they miss the faces of euphoria and they are bothered by the idea of having their mood controlled by a drug. The predominance of women among type II bipolar patients and the high number of depressive episodes in women may partially explain this phenomenon. In turn, men would be more apprehensive concerning the social and economic consequences of each episode, and this may be due to the role played by men in most societies, to the cultural expectations associated with the male role and to the fact that the probabilities of presenting with aggressive and destructive conduct is higher in men.

Contrary to what many psychiatrists may think, side effects are not one of weightier reasons to abandon treatment. In fact, in the largest survey carried out on the fears of the patients concerning medication, side effects were considered only as the seventh cause of concern regarding pharmacological treatment. Even though many psychiatrists think that lithium is one of the more frequently withdrawn treatments, its poor adherence rates are lower than those reported for other psychotropic drugs (e.g. tricyclic antidepressants).

Even though certain studies find a relationship between polymedication and poor adherence, others offer data that do not support this affirmation. The side effects may partially explain the high percentage of poor adherence recorded among the patients treated with classic neuroleptics, as described in schizophrenic patients, but most studies available in bipolar patients referred to patients treated with lithium, so that it is becoming urgent to carry out similar studies in patients treated with new drugs. Clinicians are more prone to consider that the main cause for poor adherence are the side effects and tend to overestimate them, including by ignoring the opinion of their patients. When evaluating the importance of these side effects, the psychiatrist has historically tended to place more emphasis on somatic side effects, such as tremor, nausea, or weight gain, while the patients are more worried by "psychological" effects, such as emotional flatness or the effect on cognition, or amnesic capacity. Quite probably, the fear of side effects is a better predictor of poor adherence than the side effects themselves.

It is necessary to improve the methodology of side effect studies in bipolar patients; for example, the evaluation of the presence and meaning of any drug discomfort for each patient, as part of their beliefs on health, has been so far quite variable and imprecise, and excessively depends on the variables of the patients themselves (age and personality) and their tolerance to discomfort – something that without doubt has a lot to do with their awareness of the disorder. In fact, in order to explain non-adherence, even more important than side effects themselves could be the *overestimation of side effects*: patients would be unable to tolerate even minor side effects if they are not highly motivated because of their lack of a proper illness insight. The (inner) decision of being adherent to a drug consists roughly on considering benefits and risks: if a patient does not consider bipolar disorder as a devastating illness which is potentially lethal, he may overestimate apparently tolerable side effects such as moderate diarrhea or minor tremor (as opposed to the case of the cancer patient who tolerates very important and disgusting side effects for the sake of the greatest benefit: survival).

The evaluation of the severity of each side effect is another complex topic, because most scales and inventories on side effects refer only to antipsychotics. Consequently, similar scales are needed, which would include items related to the profile of tolerability to new mood stabilizers. Currently, existing studies do not include aspects on prescription, which are obviously relevant in their follow-up, such as their complexity, cost, the administration path, etc. Further studies should include these aspects in order to contribute to determining which have more weight in adherence.

Substance use is another factor associated with poor adherence. It also seems clear that comorbidity with personality disorders, and especially with histrionic disorder, is a very solid predictor of poor adherence.

Most studies show that the number of hospitalizations is higher for patients who comply poorly, even though they have not experienced a higher number of episodes. This makes us think that – if we consider that the evolution of bipolar patients who comply poorly is worse – it is not so much because the episodes are more frequent, but because they are more severe, and makes hospitalization necessary more often.

Cognitive dysfunctions and neuropsychological deficits may be related to therapeutic adherence, and this is an area of great interest for future studies.

## The future

Extensively informing our patients about their disorder and its treatment is part of our clinical responsibility. Such simple acts as providing written information, either in the form of brochures or small monographs may help them better understand their disorder and, therefore, facilitate treatment. It is also the responsibility of the clinician to inform patients about what they should expect from a certain treatment, avoiding the creation of false-cure expectations, which, once frustrated, usually lead to the abandonment of the treatment, and about its costs and benefits. It is also necessary to teach them to handle the complicated concept of chronicity, inform them of the importance of regular habits, etc., and especially alert them to the risks of poor adherence.

The future emergence of new medications with much more acceptable tolerance profiled in classic medications, such as antidepressants, anticonvulsants and antipsychotics, will certainly be very important in improving adherence in future years, since it will help comply with therapy of all those patients whose poor adhesion is mainly due to the fear of undesirable effects. It is the responsibility of the pharmaceutical companies to understand the demand of their market, our patients, and adapt their drugs – certainly efficacious – to a format that enhances adherence.

Finally, it is highly important to identify in time the poorly compliant patient, since we have several mechanisms that can help us to improve treatment adherence.

## Session 7

# Treatment I: Mood stabilizers

## Goal

The objective of this session is to inform our patients the various types of mood stabilizers, their differences and specific indications, and their advantages and side effects. It is very important not to ignore this last part, since the patients may feel cheated if we only talk about the positive aspects of pharmacological treatment. The final objective of this session and of the entire Unit 2 is to improve adherence.

## Procedure

- After initial and formal conversation, we will ask the volunteers to present their own life charts or ones invented by them. It is to be expected that a commented presentation of a life chart will take about 15 min, so that it is advisable to make a maximum of two presentations per session.
- Next, we can start discussing the topic of the session. Taking into account that this is the first session we dedicate to drugs, we must first answer a series of questions or fears, which certain patients have about psychotropic drugs; we must make it very clear that psychotropic drugs are not addictives – except for benzodiazepines, if not properly used; that they do not "brainwash" or destroy the mind; that most of them are not stimulants; that they are not drugs "for weak people"; and that their purpose is not under any circumstance to replace the will of those who take them. Thus, we tackle at once the entire black legend surrounding psychotropic drugs.
- When entering the session, the patients would have delivered their homework on mood-stabilizing drugs. While one of the co-therapists is leading the group during the presentation of the life charts, we will have marked the most important assignments in our patients' homework and we will

discuss them during the session (always maintaining the anonymity of the comments).

- We must start by clearly differentiating what a mood-stabilizing drug is good for and what an antidepressant or antimanics are good for, and we would pay special emphasis on the preventive properties of stabilizers.
- We can continue the session by asking how many of our patients took a certain mood stabilizer at any time in their life and based on that, prepare a frequency table on the blackboard. This will serve for the members of the group to actually understand that all bipolar patients take some type of mood stabilizer, that the treatment combined with several mood stabilizers is very frequent and that in practice this treatment is different for each patient, in other words, it is tailored. This personalization contradicts the antipsychiatrist myth according to which clinicians treat patients as numbers. To us, as therapists, it can be useful to know which is the most commonly used mood stabilizer among the members of a certain group and, therefore, adapt our approach to the specific needs of the group members.
- We can write lists of side effects on the blackboard and discuss their frequency and their actual severity, in addition to certain tricks to make these side effects more bearable (e.g. a change in diet for the patients who suffer from diarrhea caused by lithium). It is extremely profitable to let the patients share their tricks themselves, so the therapist must stand aside of the discussion (because the patient would not consider "true" a very practical example coming from someone that, for example, had never suffered from tremor).
- Next, we will present the content of the material of the session and will start a round of questions and discussion.
- We will close the session by delivering the material and homework, and reminding the group that the patients who wish may present their life chart in the next session.

## Useful tips

- It is not infrequent that some of our patients think that psychiatrists have economic interest in prescribing psychotropic drugs and that part of their monthly salary depends on the number of prescriptions ordered, or that they give in to the pressure of the pharmaceutical companies. It is extremely useful to discuss these topics openly and use examples, such as that of lithium carbonate – a drug whose marketing is not particularly profitable for any company due to its low price, in spite of the fact that it is one of the most broadly used psychotropic drugs.

- Normally, the patients are interested in anecdotes surrounding the discovery of the mood-stabilizing properties of lithium salts, a discovery which goes back to 1949 and which is owed to the Australian physician, John Cade. A curious piece of information that is highly positive to reduce the stigma is that the person who was most responsible for the spreading of the use of lithium in bipolar disorders, the late Danish professor, Mogens Schou, had several persons suffering from bipolar disorders among his close family members. There is an anecdote about bipolar disorders that shows that, even though its treatment is certainly modern, its history is lengthy. This is the story of the treatments received by Ferdinand VI, the Spanish King who suffered from bipolar disorder (for more information, see Bibliography), and who underwent a great variety of therapies (Table 8; we can discuss the list in the table during the session). The fact that the disorder is very old is of interest to our patients and draws their attention, while at the same time, it makes many of them feel lucky and think "with the bad luck of having the disease like this, I was lucky to be born in a place and time when the disorder can be treated."

- One of the mistaken ideas that are rather common among our bipolar patients is to believe that the bipolar disorder is a "lack of lithium in the blood." This is an obviously false myth, but we must explain it to all our patients because it has become quite popular among the persons who suffer from bipolar disorders and even among non-specialist professionals.

- We must allow some of our patients to declare themselves in favor of certain antipharmacologic approach, since this position is quite frequent in society; in most cases, the group itself criticizes this type of position and claims the benefits of taking the medication. The professional should not adopt an excessively belligerent attitude toward the patient who makes this antipsychiatrist declaration, because this attitude could cause them to feel excluded from the group rather than included (inclusion is actually our intent), and facilitate their abandonment of the treatment.

- Concerning the topic of resistance to lithium induced by the sudden interruption in taking the medication, we can discuss it mutually, as if lithium

**Table 8.** Treatments tried by or prescribed to his Majesty Fernando VI
(1713–1759) by his personal physician, Dr. Andreu Piquer Arrufat

*Donkey's milk*
*Syrup of cochlear and water pimpernel*
*Broth with turtles, frogs, veal, and vipers*
*Enemas*
*Lime blossom and cherry infusion*
*Mother of pearl powder*
*Fumitory*
*Head baths*
*Gelatin of deer antler and young viper*
*Violets*
*Diet*
*Syrup of heliotrope scorzonera*
*Anise*
*Agrimony*

were a somewhat begrudging friend who may fail us in the future if we fail
it now.

## Patient material

We call mood stabilizers the drugs designed to maintain mood stability.
Bipolar patients need to take this type of drugs during their entire lives, and
their purpose is not only to avoid new episodes from taking place, but also
to reduce the severity and duration of a hypothetical new relapse.

Among mood stabilizers, the mostly indicated drug for the treatment of a
"pure" bipolar disorder, without any other type of complication, is certainly
*lithium*. Lithium has a strong preventive action, especially regarding manic
episodes, and also helps reduce the mood instability that affects many
patients between episodes. On the other hand, we must stress its usefulness
in *preventing suicide*; however, the sudden withdrawal of this drug may precipitate a relapse, so discontinuation – when decided by the psychiatrist –
should always be gradual. Abandoning the treatment suddenly and without
following the indications of the psychiatrist may be the cause of a future

resistance to the drug; in other words, quite probably it will not work when we resume the treatment.

The most frequent side effects of lithium are *tremor* (especially in the first weeks), *diarrhea*, increase in the need to urinate, to ingest liquids and *liquid retention*. More infrequent are acne and gastrointestinal upset.

The rest of the drugs used as mood stabilizers are generally anticonvulsants; that is, drugs indicated for the treatment of epilepsy; this does not mean that the bipolar disorder is a disorder that is "close" to epilepsy, even though they may share certain psychobiological mechanisms. Among the anticonvulsant mood stabilizers used, the main ones are *valproate, carbamazepine, oxcarbazepine,* and *lamotrigine.*

Valproate is an efficient drug to maintain euthymia, and it has a great antimanic action. It may also be efficient in the treatment of rapid cycling in mixed phases. Among its side effects, the main ones are weight increase and, more rarely, the change of hair texture or hair loss.

Another much used mood stabilizer is carbamazepine, which has been efficient in preventing relapses in bipolar disorders, including in cases of rapid cycling. It is also a good drug to treat impulsiveness. In general, carbamazepine is not associated with significant side effects, even though in certain cases it may cause vision problems (diplopia or double vision), fatigue and difficulty urinating. In exceptional cases it causes a drop in the blood sodium levels (hyponatremia). If this complication emerges, the psychiatrist must stop the drug. Without doubt, this is a very efficacious drug, but with many interactions to other drugs, so that if patients take it, they must always let their physician know when the physician prescribes a new drug. An interaction that must always be taken into account is that produced in patients who take oral contraceptives (popularly known as "The pill"), because carbamazepine reduces the efficacy of these drugs and, therefore, the protection against pregnancy is no longer complete. Oxcarbazepine is an evolved form of carbamazepine which, although it has less side effects, is also associated with the risk of hyponatremia (drop in blood sodium levels).

Lamotrigine is the most efficient drug in preventing depressive episodes, but less efficient in the prevention of manic or mixed episodes. The most common side effect of lamotrigine is the emergence of an allergic reaction on the skin (red spots that burn, known as exanthema or skin rash), which is not severe in most cases and is avoided if the dose of the drug is increased slowly until reaching the desired dose. If the spots or pimples appear on mucosa (e.g. on the lips), we must immediately consult a psychiatrist because it may be a more serious complication.

Another drug used as mood stabilizer, levothyroxin, is especially efficacious to treat rapid cycling and in cases of hyperthyroidism.

A certain atypical antipsychotic (e.g. olanzapine) may be very appropriate as maintenance drugs, especially to prevent mania, and have the obvious advantage that if a mixed hypomanic or manic phase begins, it will not be necessary to change the treatment and it would be sufficient to increase the dose of olanzapine. One of the main side effects of olanzapine is weight gain.

Fortunately, psycho-pharmacology is an area that experiences constant progress and it is foreseeable that the list will soon increase.

---

**Assignment 6**

Have you taken or are you taking any antimanic (haloperidol, clotiapine, olanzapine, risperidone, quetiapine, ziprasidone)? What do you think they are good for? Do they cause you any discomfort?

# Session 8

# Treatment II: Antimanic drugs

## Goal

The objective of the eighth session is to give the group updated information on the pharmacological treatment of the manic and hypomanic phases in order to improve patient adherence in these phases, since it is usually deficient.

## Procedure

- As usual, we will start the group with a brief informal conversation, after which we will ask (two) volunteers to present a life chart.
- Next, we will ask our patients about the use of various antimanic drugs ("How many of you had to take olanzapine?" "How many have taken risperidone?" etc.), on their indication ("Do you remember at what point they were prescribed to you?" "Were you in a manic or depressed phase?") and about adherence ("How many of you stopped taking it without the physician telling you to?"). We can make a list of usage frequencies on the blackboard, as we did in the session on mood stabilizers.
- At this point, the patients probably have already introduced the topic of antimanic drugs and their advantages and inconvenience, and we can start presenting all material. From time to time, we will interrupt our explanation to ask the patients about the side effects of a certain drug, if they had taken it, and thus make our presentation more interactive.
- We switch to a phase of questions and discussion and, after delivering the material and homework, we close the session.

## Useful tips

- It is appropriate to update often the information we give the patients in the written material. We all know that one of the areas of psycho-pharmacology which has most advanced recently is that of antipsychotics/antimanic drugs, and it is important to keep our patients well informed about all drugs they potentially may take, including those that are starting to be marketed and which, even though their using treating mania has not been approved, are starting to be used by the clinician's. If we do not update our information in time, the patient may doubt the truthfulness and validity of our entire approach.

- The fact that most antimanic drugs are antipsychotics, broadly used in the treatment of schizophrenia, usually confuses patients about the nature of their own disorder and makes them wonder to what extent the two disorders are "twin disorders." This point must be clarified during our explanation, reminding the patients that, even though the two disorders share certain symptoms and part of their pharmacological treatment, it does not mean that they are the same disorder.

- A common question of the patients is "What happens if we do not treat mania?" "How long can it last?" Our answer must be firm and decisive and we must emphasize all sort of risks associated with mania (deterioration of work, social, affective and academic life, and more cognitive impairment in the long term), remind them that the duration of the depressive shift is generally proportionate to the intensity of the manic symptoms and stress that mania is "fun" only in its first stages, and not for all patients.

- Since this is one of the objectives of our intervention, it is fundamental to place special stress both on the preventive aspects (among them, not abandoning the treatment from the start) as well as the therapeutic aspects, properly speaking. This usually gives our patients a feeling of better control over their disorder.

## Patient material

The treatment of a manic or hypomanic phase would greatly depend on the intensity of the symptoms. The *early identification* of this type of decompensation is essential to prevent its intensity from becoming too strong and, consequently, to avoid hospitalization and avoiding an especially aggressive treatment, with all side effects it implies, in spite of more recent pharmacological progress. In most cases, early identification will prevent a new episode that may seriously alter our lives. The manic episodes may be successfully treated only with psychotropic drugs, while the psychological intervention would be more indicated to prevent and facilitate early identification. Consequently, it is senseless to try to treat mania with psychotherapy. Progress in the research of psychotropic drugs has allowed us to increase the efficacy of the new antimanic drugs and reduce their side effects. There are several types of antimanic drugs, and some of them are described below:

- *Neuroleptics or classic antipsychotics.* Classic neuroleptics have been for decades the absolutely necessary tool in the successful therapy of any manic picture, and in spite of the fact that in many places they were pushed aside by the new version, atypical or second generation antipsychotics (about which we will speak later on) even to date, they are the most direct and rapid drugs for the treatment of mania. As the name indicates, they are efficacious in treating the psychotic symptoms, for example, delirium and hallucinations (which are not infrequent in mania), they help reduce grandiose thinking, successfully control agitation and irritability, normalize the course of thought (i.e. slow down the accelerated thinking that is typical for mania and certain hypomanias) and their content, which are strange and inadequate ideas. Since they were replaced by atypical antimanic drugs, most classic neuroleptics are no longer used today, although some continue being used broadly due to their quick action, which has not yet been reached by the newer drugs; this is the case of haloperidol. The simple administration of a few drops of haloperidol for a few days sometimes suffices to slow down a new episode, provided we detect it in time. Its most frequent side effects are muscle rigidity, tremor, the emergence of tics, a feeling of sadness, restlessness in the legs (akathisia), and various anticholinergic effects (dry mouth, etc.). The possibility for the emergence of these side effects, which are quite reversible a few days after stopping the drug, makes the psychiatrist always choose the smallest possible dose. On the other hand, most of these side effects disappear or are alleviated with the administration of anti-Parkinson drugs.
- *New antimanic drugs.* The new antimanic drugs, or atypical antipsychotics, are drugs marketed especially in the last decade, in order to match or exceed the therapeutic properties of haloperidol and improve their side effect profile. In other words, these are drugs as or more efficacious as haloperidol and clotiapine, but they cause much or less discomfort. The

efficacy of most of these atypical antipsychotics has been demonstrated in maintenance treatment, and for this reason, they may be used at low doses as mood stabilizers (in general, in combination with a classic mood stabilizer), to avoid manic relapses and the emergence of psychotic symptoms. Some of them such as olanzapine or quetiapine has shown to be efficacious for the depressive phase of the disorder. Following are among the main atypical antipsychotics:

– *Olanzapine.* This is one of the new antimanic drugs about which we have more information, coming from rigorous scientific carried out in thousands of patients throughout the world. It is a highly efficacious drug in the treatment of mania, regardless of its subtype (euphoric or dysphoric), and quite adequate for maintenance treatment; it can also help in the treatment of certain depressive phases. It causes very few side effects, and in general, is very well tolerated by all patients. The only potential problem is that it usually causes weight gain.

– *Quetiapine.* This is perhaps the atypical antimanic drug that produces less side effects: less weight increase than risperidone and olanzapine and practically no sexual dysfunction. In certain cases, it may reduce blood pressure so that it is not indicated in hypotensive patients. Another common side effect is sedation. It might be also useful as a mood stabilizer and in some types of bipolar depressions.

– *Risperidone.* This is another widely used drug, very efficacious antimanic and a powerful antipsychotic. It is also used in maintenance treatment at low doses and it is especially efficacious in preventing rapid cycling. Its side effects are similar to those of haloperidol, even though much milder. It produces less weight gains than olanzapine, but may cause reversible hormonal changes, such as an increase in prolactin and sexual dysfunction (e.g. erection problems or anorgasmia).

– *Others.* Little by little, new atypical antipsychotics are being introduced in the treatment of mania, such as ziprasidone or aripiprazol, and this will allow many patients who perhaps so far have not adequately responded to the available drugs to benefit from adequate treatment. These two newer drugs are expected to cause less sedation than the existing ones.

• *Benzodiazepines.* The most broadly used hypnotic (drug to facilitate sleep) in the treatment of manic and hypomanic phases is clonazepam, quite efficacious in patients presenting with a lot of anxiety, agitation, irritability, or insomnia. Other drugs such as lorazepam or diazepam may contribute to the treatment to the extent that it improves sleep and reduces anxiety, but it is absolutely not indicated to treat the manic picture only with these drugs.

- *Others.* The increase in the dose of mood stabilizer (lithium, valproate, carbamazepine, or oxcarbazepine) may also be efficacious in the treatment of moderate mania, but the slow action of these drugs makes them inappropriate in most occasions. They are indicated, however, in the first episodes with mild or moderate intensity. Electroconvulsive therapy (ECT) is a very safe and hugely efficacious treatment, absolutely necessary in certain special cases (e.g. pregnant patients, drug-resistant mania, etc.).

As we can see, there is a variety of treatments available to face the manic or hypomanic phase, even though prevention is always the best treatment.

---

**Assignment 7**

Have you taken or are you taking any antidepressant (fluoxetine, paroxetine, venlafaxine, citalopram, clomipramine, imipramine, or others)? What do you think they are good for? Do they cause you any discomfort?

# Treatment III: Antidepressants

## Goal

The objective of this ninth session is to inform the group about the pharmacological treatment of the depressive and mixed phases. As already happened in the clinical section (see p. 85), in the session on depression information on mixed phases is included for purely logistical reasons of time availability, although the treatment of the mixed phases is more similar to the treatment of mania than to the treatment of depression.

## Procedure

- As has been usual in the last sessions, we will start the session with an informal conversation after which we will ask (two) volunteers to present their life chart.
- After completing the presentation of the life charts, we will ask the patients which they believe is the conduct to adopt in the event of depression, their opinion on the use of various antidepressant drugs and adherence, and what they think about the possible role of a psychological treatment. Again, we can make a list of use frequencies of antidepressants on the blackboard, as we did in the previous two sessions.
- Before starting to explain at length the treatment of depression, we will insist on the difference between depression and sadness as a normal emotion and will specify that sadness, like any other regular mood, cannot and must not be "treated," since it is not a disease.
- Then, we will present the material of the session.
- The session is closed as always after the questions round and discussion, and after delivering the material and the homework.

## Useful tips

- Once again, we must constantly update the written material we provide to the patients.
- An aspect that must be especially stressed concerns the risks of self-medication with antidepressants, since many bipolar patients misuse these drugs. We must stress and emphasize the medical risks, the risks of shifts, rapid cycling, interaction and course worsening caused by this misuse.
- It is very important for the patient to get the message that the pharmacological treatment is personalized depending on the needs, background and characteristics of each patient, and therefore it is difficult to find two identical patterns. Many patients ask what are the differences between various drugs in the same family (e.g. the selective serotonin reuptake inhibitors, SSRIs). Besides explaining the subtle differences between the various drugs, we must insist on prior response as an indicator of therapeutic response.
- As to the topic of the usefulness of psychological treatments, it is important to tell the patients that they do not work in any case as monotherapy in bipolar disorders; even though the therapeutic efficacy of some of these psychological treatments improving some symptoms of bipolar depression has been demonstrated, especially in mild–moderate depressions or in patients with great potential for shifts, or also in type III bipolar patients, they must always be combined with mood-stabilizer treatment and many times with an antidepressant. We remind them that, to date, there are clinical trials with partially good results in bipolar depression only for two psychological treatments, namely cognitive therapy and interpersonal therapy of social rhythms.
- At the end of the session, the patient must have understood that not just any psychological treatment is efficacious in tackling bipolar depression, and that some would even be contraindicated. It is important for the patient not to interpret our argument as a "defense of the paradigm," and therefore we must briefly explain the difference between science, beliefs and opinions, and place each psychological treatment in its appropriate place based on the literature available to date. This is a topic which will be broadly treated during the session dedicated to alternative treatments (see p. 135).

## Patient material

Unlike the treatment of manic episodes, in which antipsychotics are practically the only possible treatment, we have several alternatives to treat depressive phases:

- *Antidepressants.* Antidepressants are efficacious enough to treat bipolar depression. The doses and side effects are similar to those of their use in unipolar depression, with the exception that, in patients with bipolar disorders they are associated with the risk of inducing a manic or mixed episode, or one including rapid cycling. Because of this, the psychiatrist is cautious when prescribing them. They must always be administered in combination with a mood stabilizer. Among the most broadly used antidepressants, we find the following:

  – *Tricyclic antidepressants.* They have constituted a main weapon of pharmacotherapy against depression for almost 30 years, since they were among the first psychotropic drugs discovered. They are probably the most rapid and efficacious drugs in the treatment of bipolar depression, but they also produce more side effects or discomfort, and are associated with a higher risk of causing a change of phase. They tend to produce sedation in most patients, even though some feel stimulated. They often cause hypotension, which tends to be postural. Sometimes there is weight gain during the treatment. The most broadly used are imipramine and clomipramine.

  – *Selective serotonin reuptake inhibitors (SSRIs).* These are drugs practically as efficacious as the tricyclics, but cause less side effects and have less potential to induce mania or hypomania, so that currently they are a group of drugs used broadly to treat bipolar depression. Quite often their side effects are reduced to slight digestive discomfort at the beginning of the treatment and, occasionally, sexual dysfunction. Some of the most used SSRIs are fluoxetine and paroxetine, which are highly indicated in depressions with a large anxiety component, and finally sertraline and citalopram.

  – *Monoamine oxidase inhibitors (MAOIs).* Their use is relatively limited, in spite of their great efficacy, because they interact with many commonly used drugs (e.g. those used to treat a cold). In addition, they force the patient to follow a special diet, since they also interact with fermented foods with high tyramine content and may cause a hypertensive crisis, cerebral hemorrhage or infarction if this rule is not followed. Consequently, the patient who takes MAOIs must not eat any of the following foods: sausage, fermented cheeses, wine and beer, pickles, foods in vinegar or marinade, most canned foods, avocados figs, bananas, caviar, prawns, dried fish, smoked meat or fish, and precooked dishes. Some of the most common MAOIs are tranylcypromine and phenelzine. Moclobemide is an MAOI that presents less risk of drug and food interactions.

– *Selective serotonin and noradrenaline reuptake inhibitors (SSNRIs).* These are the most recent antidepressants. Their effect may be more potent than SSRIs; they may be considered equally as efficacious as tricyclics and are also associated with less side effects, even though their potential to induce mania may be higher than the SSRIs. The SSNRI currently available is venlafaxine. Another mixed action drug (noradrenergic and serotonergic) is mirtazapine, which seems to be less effective and induces serious weight gain and sedation.

• *Lamotrigine.* This drug, which is not exactly an antidepressant, was already discussed in the session on stabilizers (see Session 7, p. 115). Its antidepressant action is usually slow, especially because the physician must increase the dose quite slowly to avoid the emergence of side effects, but it is very safe because its potential to induce mania is practically zero.

• *Electroconvulsive therapy (ECT).* It is highly efficacious in the case of more inhibited depressions or those more resistant to drug treatment. We have already indicated that this therapy is very safe (see p. 121).

• *Psychological therapies.* The only psychological therapies whose efficacy in the treatment of bipolar depression has been demonstrated are cognitive therapy and interpersonal therapy, which are combined with the administration of antidepressants and always with stabilizers. It has not been demonstrated that psychoanalysis has any usefulness in the treatment of bipolar disorders.

---

### Assignment 8

If you take lithium, valproic acid, or carbamazepine, Do you know how often you must have a control test? Do you know why they are needed? Do you know what are the ideal levels of these drugs in the blood? Have you ever had excessively high lithium levels? What happened?

# Session 10

# Plasma levels of mood stabilizers

## Goal

The objective of this session is for the patient to understand the need for periodic tests in order to determine serum levels. Many patients do not do these serum determinations regularly, either because they forget, because they do not understand their importance or because they are afraid of needles. Others, on the contrary, overestimate the need/usefulness of these tests and give them diagnostic or prognostic value concerning the evolution of their disorder. This tenth session is intended to focus on and stress the importance of serum determinations of mood stabilizers.

## Procedure

- As usual, the session starts with the presentation of two life charts.
- After these presentations, we may start asking our patients how many of them take lithium, valproate, and carbamazepine and how many of them have had a lithium, valproate, or carbamazepine plasma concentration taken in the last half year. If the number does not match, we will ask why some of them did not have the test. Later we can ask whether they know why they must have regular determinations of their levels of mood stabilizers and we will review the homework.
- We will present the material of the session and will open the round of questions and the discussion.
- We will deliver the material and the assignment and will end the session.

## Useful tips

- Most of our explanation must be focused on the importance of lithium plasma concentration, the same as most of the explanation in the seventh session was focused on lithium, since it is even today the most broadly used stabilizer – at least in Europe.

- One of the most common mistakes made by our patients, as already indicated, is to think that the cause of the bipolar disorder is related to the low level of lithium in the blood, and therefore they give lithium plasma concentration diagnostic value. This belief is quite widespread among our patients, partly due to deficient information provided by many non-specialized physicians. We must make it quite clear to the members of the group that the value of lithium plasma concentration is that it serves to control the treatment and to make sure that lithium does not reach toxic levels. We must also clarify that if we do a lithium plasma concentration in a person who does not take lithium, whether or not bipolar, the levels will be undetectable, and this does not indicate the presence of any pathology.

- Concerning the importance of salt in the diet, it must be explained to our patients that they may follow a low-sodium (not no-sodium) diet, provided it is a medical necessity, and provided they have a lithium plasma concentration after the first days of following such a diet. This lithium plasma concentration will serve to prove that there is no increase in lithium levels that may imply a risk. In turn, we must reassure all patients concerning subtle and daily changes in salt in the foods, since such changes do not imply any risk.

- The risk of lithium poisoning due to dehydration must be explicitly discussed during the session, because there are many cases of patients that start going to the sauna with a certain frequency while taking lithium and, as a consequence, they experience the sudden emergence of side effects due to the increase in lithium levels. There was even one female patient who started going to the sauna to calm "a constant anxiety that made my hands tremble." Obviously, and given that the trembling was associated with lithium, the more sauna she had, the more she trembled. The patient did not know the relationship between the sauna and lithium levels and decided to increase the frequency of her sauna sessions because she felt increasingly "nervous" (she trembled more). Her condition could have ended with severe poisoning if this conduct has not been detected in a timely fashion.

## Patient material

As indicated in previous sessions, it is very important to know the levels reached by mood-stabilizing drugs (lithium, valproate, carbamazepine, oxcarbazepine) in the blood, to make sure that:

1　The drug reaches a sufficiently high concentration to be therapeutic, that is to be useful.
2　The concentration of the drug is not excessive, since at high-enough levels it may be toxic.
3　The patient is taking the medication correctly.

The frequency of the tests will vary. In the beginning, we must do many, until we find the optimal serum level, which corresponds to the maximum therapeutic effect of the medication and the lowest number of side effects. Once this level is established the psychiatrist will request a level determination in the following situations:

1　Routine control every 6 months.
2　Whenever the dose of mood stabilizer is modified or other drugs that may interact with them are modified.
3　When it is suspected that the patient is taking the drug incorrectly.
4　When poisoning or too high levels are suspected.

In general, we will suspect lithium poisoning in the presence of symptoms such as intense tremor, vertigo, vomiting, convulsions, vision problems, intense diarrhea, movement coordination problems, or confusional states. Carbamazepine, oxcarbazepine, and valproate have lower toxic potential than lithium.

Lithium levels in the blood must range between 0.4 and 1.4 mEq/l: below these levels it would have no therapeutic effect and above them the risk of poisoning would be very high. The levels of carbamazepine must be between 5 and 15 mg/ml and those of valproate between 50 and 100 mg/ml.

We must take into account that lithium is a salt and therefore its levels may oscillate depending on various factors, such as for example hyposodic diet (low-salt diet) or in periods of severe dehydration (e.g. due to saunas or viral infections that cause fever or vomiting, making a physical effort that makes one sweat profusely). Consequently, patients who take lithium must avoid sudden changes in the salt content of their diet. This is also recommendable for patients treated with carbamazepine or oxcarbazepine because of the risk of hyponatremia.

The determination of serum levels must be done 10 days after changing the dose, because within a shorter period of time the dose change is not reflected in the test. The day of the test it is necessary to avoid taking the immediately prior mood-stabilizer intake, to avoid altering the test results.

---

**Assignment 9**

How do you believe your bipolar disorder affects your decision to have or not to have children? What are your concerns related to the future of your children?

---

# Session 11

## Pregnancy and genetic counseling

### Goal

This session is especially addressed to our female patients, since its objective is to tackle the problematic relationship between psychotropic drugs and pregnancy. Given that this knowledge area has evolved significantly in recent years, we had to update the contents of the session several times; in the first groups, 10 years ago, we gave our patients instructions about how to plan a pregnancy based on the treatment with lithium salts. With the data we had available at that time, we considered that lithium always had to be stopped before conception, so that the pregnancies had to be perfectly well programmed in moments of stability. Subsequently, this message has become milder because the studies on the teratogenic risk of various psychotropic drugs – including lithium – do not offer such dramatic data, and the session is now focused on offering the patients sufficient information so that at a given time they may make the most suitable decision. The fundamental message of the session is that in all events, the patient must always consult her psychiatrist before deciding to become pregnant, in order to be able to have rigorous control along with her gynecologist. In the first years of the psychoeducation program, certain male patients requested permission to be absent from the session because they considered that it was not useful to them. The truth is that during the session there is a lot of discussion about the heritability of the bipolar disorder and the capacity of a person who suffers from the disorder to act as a father or mother, so we consider that the topic is of interest for all our patients.

### Procedure

- After the initial informal conversation, we will ask like always (two) volunteers to present their life chart.

- We may ask how many of our female patients have children and what is the attitude of their psychiatrist concerning medication during pregnancy. Generally, this is useful to introduce the topic.
- We will facilitate the debate about whether or not a person who suffers from bipolar disorder may take the responsibility implied in the role of father or mother, and about what it would mean to each of them if their child had bipolar disorder. We can get inspiration from the assignments done by the patients. We will allow this debate to take a great part of the session, since in the end it is a crucial issue concerning the acceptance of the disorder.
- We will present the rest of the material, we will deliver it together with the homework and we will close the session.

## Useful tips

- Concerning postpartum episodes, we must make it quite clear that their origin is psychobiological, that they are related to a sudden drop in estrogens and other organic changes, and not psycho-social factors of a change of role. Clarifying these matters allows us to stress further the biological character of the disorder.
- The final decision as to whether or not the patient will take medication during pregnancy is always up to her; the professional can only inform and facilitate pro or con arguments. Certain patients view this type of advice as an interference. During the group sessions, we will provide only general information and will avoid commenting on concrete cases, in addition to inviting the patients to discuss the topic with their psychiatrist.
- In this session certain traumatic aspects appear or are appealed, related to what the disorder means or represents for each person, especially when certain patients, generally those who have had a particularly negative experience of bipolar disorder, make affirmations such as "I will never have a child; I do not want to destroy his life with this disorder" or "I will never forgive myself if my child inherits the disorder"; other patients, however, may feel offended by these phrases pronounced by their group mates and even reject them during the session, since their experience of the disorder is not so dramatic. ("I did not choose to have this disorder,

but I am getting along well with treatment. It is also no drama if my child inherits it.") The therapist must bring up this discussion in this session and in others, since it is enriching for the patients and allows them to explore positions concerning the disorder that may improve their acceptance. In principle, if the discussion follows the rules of mutual respect, it is better for the therapist not to intervene or, in any event, to intervene as an arbitrator. The therapist must not under any circumstances *take sides* since the patients may have difficulty accepting a person who is not ill speaking about how a patient feels about their disorder.

- The treatment of bipolar disorders has experienced a spectacular evolution in the last 15 years, and it may be foreseen that this evolution will be even more spectacular in the next 15 years. Stressing it may help certain patients to undramatize the possibility that their future child would present with bipolar disorders in 20 years.

## Patient material

One of the topics that most worries our patients is everything related to children. In today's session we will try to answer questions such as "Can I have children if I have bipolar disorder?", "Will my child have bipolar disorder?", or "Must I stop taking my medication if I want to become pregnant?"

Many couples in which one of the members has a chronic disease of genetic origin such as bipolar disorders discuss the possibility of having children, but feel doubt given that there is a possibility that the children will also have the same disorder. This probability will depend on highly varied factors, including the number of family members with the same disease, the number of children, the subtype of the disorder, whether the person affected is the future father or the future mother, and even luck. Other factors that have a very big weight are obviously the paternal or maternal vocation, the idea a person has of his or her disorder, the family context, and the severity of the disorder, since a decompensated bipolar disorder is probably incompatible with performing the obligations of a father or mother.

In general, we can affirm that the risk that the children of bipolar disorder patients will also have the disorder is higher than in the children of those who do not have it. In any case, the risk for the children of those affected is *about 20%*, which means that the child has more possibilities not to have the disorder

(80%) than to have it (20%). This risk is much higher if both the father and the mother have bipolar disorder or another affective disorder. It must be stressed that we do not always speak of immediate inheritance, because sometimes the disorder skips one or two generations, and the disorder is not always inherited with the same intensity or the same form: a type I bipolar disorder father may have a child with type II bipolar disorder, for example.

It is highly recommendable that, if a bipolar patient wants to have a child, *she must duly plan the pregnancy*, since there is a certain risk that some of the most broadly used medications to treat bipolar disorders would cause malformations in the fetus. We must consequently consider the possibility of stopping these medications without omitting to take into account the risk of relapse, since a relapse during pregnancy makes it difficult and is also undesirable. The bipolar patient who wishes to become pregnant must tell her psychiatrist in advance so that the latter starts the progressive removal of the drugs he finds appropriate, or even to indicate what is the best time according to the clinical evolution; ideally, the best is for the pregnancy to coincide with a moment of stability, both because it is a very important decision that must be made responsibly, and this rarely happens when the patient is in mania or depression phase, and because the reduction in the dose of medication implies a risk of relapse which we cannot add to the risk of having suffered an episode recently.

Lithium has been associated with an increase in the risk of emergence of certain congenital malformations such as *Ebstein's anomaly* (heart malformation), but it is a relatively low risk. If the psychiatrist and the patient agree to remove lithium temporarily, such removal must be done progressively throughout the 6 months prior to the pregnancy. Lithium is usually reintroduced without too many risks starting in the second trimester of pregnancy, since the teratogenic risk is significant, especially when the fetus forms, that is during the first trimester. On the other hand, the psychiatrist may choose drugs with lower teratogenic risk or, in the event of a relapse, opt for treatment with electroconvulsive therapy, which is safe both for the patient and for the fetus. Valproate is associated with a certain risk of spina bifida in the fetus, which is somewhat lower for carbamazepine. In both the cases, it is highly recommendable to also take folic acid before pregnancy.

If the removal of lithium is synonymous with an immediate relapse, it may be maintained throughout the pregnancy, controlling the risk of malformations with periodic ultrasounds. If a malformation is detected, the woman may decide on voluntary interruption of the pregnancy, if she so wishes.

In any case, the phase of the highest risk of relapse is not the pregnancy but postpartum. Concretely, 50% of untreated patients present with a manic or depressive episode after giving birth, caused by the sudden drop in estrogen. For this reason, if the treatment was interrupted it is particularly important to introduce it immediately after the birth.

As to breastfeeding, it is preferable to bottle-feed the baby and give up breastfeeding, since certain medications (e.g. lithium) may pass from the blood to the mother's milk and constitute a risk of poisoning for the baby.

To conclude, we will remind you that certain medications interact with oral contraceptives (*anti-baby* pills), for example carbamazepine and, to a lesser degree, oxcarbazepine, and their efficacy is reduced, so that the patients who take carbamazepine must use another type of contraceptive measures (barrier contraceptives, such as the condom or the intrauterine device (IUD)). Hormonal contraceptives may cause emotional disturbances but not decompensations.

---

**Assignment 10**

Have you ever tried to treat your disorder with a therapy or product not indicated by your psychiatrist? Why? What happened? What do you think may be the role of spiritual cure, astrology, yoga, meditation, and other alternative therapies in the treatment of a bipolar patient?

# Session 12

## Psycho-pharmacology vs. alternative therapies

### Goal

Many bipolar patients seek the help of alternative treatments (homeopathy, naturopathy, esoteric therapies, etc.) and from parascientific professionals (clairvoyant, spiritual advisors, or healers), in most cases ignoring the differences between the medical treatment of the disorder and the alternative treatments as to evidence and efficacy. The objective of this session is to explain to our patients what this difference is, what steps are followed in a treatment before its approval and why certain supposed alternative therapies do not work in the case of bipolar patients.

### Procedure

- If there are still patients who volunteer to present their life chart, we will dedicate the first 20–30 min to a couple of cases.
- Unlike the previous sessions, in Session 12 we will not start our presentation with an open question to the patients. As most of the general population does not know how the scientific method works and what a clinical study is, we will start by explaining these two issues, and this will allow us to make constant references to the scientific or non-scientific character of a certain treatment during the debate, after presenting the material of the session, without having to interrupt ourselves in order to clarify these terms to our patients.
- Based on the material of the assignments, we will facilitate the discus-sion between patients about the role of alternative therapies in bipolar disorders.
- We may choose to review the "alternative treatments" one by one or all at once. In any case, it is positive to make a distinction between those that are only innocuous and those that are damaging.

- We will present the material.
- We will deliver the material of the following session and the homework, and after that we will close the session.

## Useful tips

- In this specific session it is impossible and absurd for the therapist to claim not "to take sides," since he is clearly on one side of the discussion. In any case, it is preferable that, during the debate that is generated by this session we allow the patients themselves to argue among them, even though our position is clear. In all events, we can always point out data we consider pertinent and that are perhaps ignored by our patients.
- If there is a single patient who defends the "alternative" approach, we must try not to allow them to be isolated in the group by the mere fact that their arguments are different (even if they are clearly wrong); on the one hand, it is good to prevent the discussion from becoming too lengthy and the tone excessively harsh, and to try to close it with conciliating words without making any concession to para-scientific arguments.
- In many groups, when this session starts, the topic of religious beliefs comes up. Given that it is a delicate topic which is affectively linked to the life of many of our patients, both favorably and negatively, in this case it is better for us to tackle the topic without exposing it to excessive debate. Obviously, our answer must be that neither faith nor praying are treatments of bipolar disorder, but that they may be important for those who were already believers earlier, in spite of the fact that, in a bipolar person, it is always necessary to mistrust conversions or epiphanies because they may be the sign of the inception of an episode.
- The patients who are closest or most in favor of alternative therapies reject our arguments with anecdotes of isolated cases that had a spectacularly good response to a certain alternative intervention. We can answer this argument solidly in front of the group only if we had previously explained clearly what the scientific method is and what a clinical trial is.
- Certain patients ask us whether they may take a certain alternative treatment together with their standard pharmacological treatment. In general there is no medical problem to prevent it, but we must explain to the patient that it is counterproductive to complain on the one hand that "one

is taking too many drugs" and on the other hand, to follow a treatment that has no guarantee whatsoever.

## Patient material

So far we have reviewed the pharmacological treatment of bipolar disorders. Before being marketed, all these treatments have been submitted to highly rigorous studies that include animal investigation in the lab and testing on volunteers, both healthy and sick, whose purpose is to prove the safety, tolerance, and efficacy of the new drugs.

As to safety and tolerance, a drug is safe when it is proven that it cannot damage the patient who takes it, and it is considered tolerable when the therapeutic effects may be worthy compared to the side effects. This is the case of lithium which, even though it may produce certain discomfort to those who take it (tremor, diarrhea, etc.) is perfectly tolerable if we compare these discomforts to the severe problems that may arise from not taking lithium: constant relapses, hospitalizations, loss of work, breakup of affective relations, suicide attempts, etc.

The third objective of clinical studies on a drug is to determine its efficacy, in other words, whether it serve to improve or eliminate the symptoms it is supposed to treat. But a drug must not only demonstrate that it is "better than nothing," but it must also demonstrate equal or higher efficacy than the drugs already used to treat a certain disease. All these studies, which come at a very high economic cost for the companies that carry them out, allow us to assure that the drugs that reach the pharmacy are authentic treatments and not fraud.

Something similar happens with psychological treatments; even though efficacy studies have less tradition in psychology than in medicine, today several studies of this type are being carried out throughout the world in order to eliminate once and for all the idea of "everything goes," so widespread among the general population concerning the psychologist. The psychotherapeutic intervention must always be based on studies demonstrating its efficacy in a significant number of patients. One must forget forever the intuitive or "magic" intervention, so popular among certain psychologists and which has caused so much damage to the profession.

Although it is very clear that any treatment may demonstrate its efficacy through the scientific method, the person who suffers from bipolar disorder or any other disorder till today must make an effort to ignore the promises of allegedly miracle cures, since there are large numbers of treatments without any scientific basis which are presented as curative but which, at best, are innocuous, and in most cases, constitute fraud that may cause severe damage to the health of the trusting patient.

A strict but valid definition of "alternative treatments" would say that they are all those that are not included in the series of therapeutic possibilities considered by the scientific community for a concrete disease. In the case of bipolar disorders, what we mean by standard treatment is most pharmacological treatments presented here and electroconvulsive therapy. Among psychological therapies, in the realm of bipolar disorders, efficacy has been demonstrated only by psychoeducation (both for patients and for family members), cognitive–behavioral therapy, and interpersonal therapy.

Concerning psychodynamic therapies, such as for example psychoanalysis, it must be said that in its time, meaning in the first half of the twentieth century, they constituted a true social and cultural revolution. However, so far not only has it not been demonstrated that they have any efficacy in the treatment of bipolar disorders (although they may be useful to elaborate on certain aspects of the personality of an individual, especially if he does not suffer any mental disorder), but also in many cases this type of therapy induces a certain worsening of the symptoms as a consequence of the high level of stress to which the patient is exposed. Most of these approaches also insist – against all scientific evidence – on the importance of understanding bipolar disorder as a consequence of the patient's emotional traumas and conflicts, ignoring the true cause of the disorder, which is biologic, inducing guilt in patients and their families and, in certain cases, attempts to stop the pharmacologic treatment which, as we already know, is indispensable in treating this disorder. All this may cause an increase in the number of patient relapses. In certain cases, perhaps it makes sense to incorporate certain classic elements from psychodynamic therapies into the standard psychological therapy, but without losing sight of the medical model.

More severe is the case of the mystical–religious–spiritual–esoteric–orientalist therapies. On the one hand, because it has not been demonstrated that they have any efficacy or usefulness and, on the other hand, because there is no need for any official degrees to practice as "therapist" in this type of allegedly curative interventions. In most cases, they are done by persons without any training in psychiatry or clinical psychology, and are a fertile ground for the practice of ignorance – in the best of cases – and charlatans. It can also not be ruled out that *a posteriori*, this type of intervention is the entry door to sect movements which basically feed on persons with some type of psychological pathology, taking advantage of their helplessness and desperation.

Concerning homeopathy and so-called natural treatments, it must be said that, for now, it has not been demonstrated that they have any efficacy in the treatment of bipolar disorders. The main advantage of these treatments is that they produce as few side effects as a glass of water, and their main problem is that their therapeutic efficacy is also similar to a glass of water, in other words, ZERO as demonstrated so far. In all events, to demonstrate the efficacy of any of these treatments, if it exists, it would be sufficient to submit them to rigorous scientific study. Without doubt, a bipolar patient treated only with homeopathy will suffer constant relapses and in addition will experience an aggravation of the evolution of the disorder.

Mental health is too serious a matter to leave it in the hands of persons with little training or treat it with products whose efficacy has not been demonstrated. Only adequate treatment with drugs and the intervention of a psychologist specialized in techniques with proven efficacy may guarantee a more positive evolution of the bipolar disorder.

---

**Assignment 11**

Have you ever stopped taking the medication without the psychiatrist telling you to do so? Describe what happened, why you stopped, and how you believe that taking the medication may harm you.

# Risks associated with treatment withdrawal

## Goal

Poor adherence is a problem that affects all medical disciplines and quite especially psychiatry. In the case of bipolar patients whose awareness of the disorder is altered, poor adherence is one of the most frequent problems and the main cause for recurrence. This session, which closes the unit of adherence improvement, is designed to fix the contents of the unit and make the patients understand the risk of relapse associated with the abandonment of the treatment.

## Procedure

- After the initial or warm-up conversation, we will review some of the life charts presented by our patients, especially those cases in which the patient abandoned the treatment at any point. We will use this to analyze what happens after abandoning the treatment, which in general is a recurrence. If we do not have enough life charts, or if poor adherence is not a relevant factor in any of them, we can use Example 4 in Session 6 (see p. 96).
- This is another one of those sessions that generate great interaction between patients. In our 10-year experience with psychoeducation groups of bipolar patients, it is a very rare group in which there is no patient who defends positions justifying poor adherence. Once again, it will be very positive if it is not the psychologist or psychiatrist who appears to be the only defender of the need to take medication, even though obviously he would already have taken this position in front of the group; it is appropriate for the patients themselves to advise good adherence.
- This session, and one of the previous ones, are rather propitious for confessions of poor adherence by the patients, which is very positive both for patients who speak sincerely and for their group mates. If this happens, we

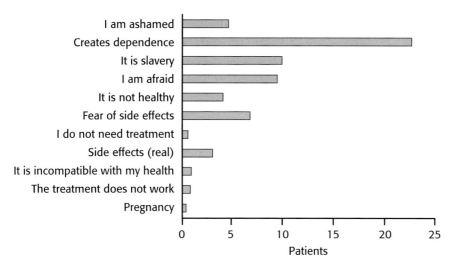

Figure 5    Result of the BEAM survey of bipolar patients on the most frequent reasons for abandoning treatment (Morselli et al., 2003).

will try to have patients explain their reasons without being interrupted by the rest of the group, and we will not adopt under any circumstances an openly critical attitude. Our first reaction must always be to thank the patient for their sincerity and for showing us enough trust to explain such a significant problem both to (we) therapists, as well as to the other members of the group. We must give them the feeling that we understand the reasons for abandoning treatment but, at the same time, issue a warning of the risk it entails and recommend that they contact their psychiatrist immediately. If we know that the psychiatrist is at the center at that precise moment, it will be very positive if one of the co-therapists organizes an unscheduled visit after contacting the psychiatrist. It is also positive for us to invite patients who abandoned their treatment at some point to describe their experiences to the group.

• Before reviewing the material of the session, it may be very useful to propose an exercise that consists of making a list, with the help of the patients, of the possible reasons of a person who suffers from bipolar disorder to abandon the treatment (Figure 5). As always, we will use the blackboard for this list.

• If we think it is appropriate, we can use some type of chart such as that in Figure 6, which illustrates the complexity of the factors associated with poor adherence.

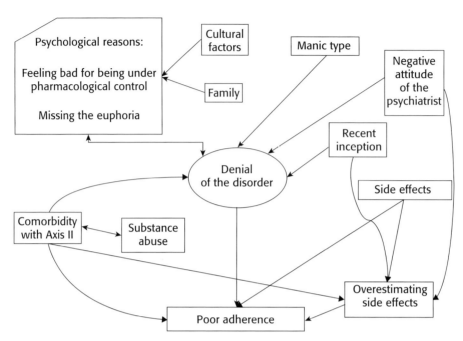

Figure 6    Factors associated with poor therapeutic adherence.

- There is also a type of participative round that is extremely useful for our patients and at the same time is pleasant: this is the round of "tricks not to forget the medication," or in other words, how each patient organizes their daily intake of prescribed treatment. This exercise helps the therapists to learn new methods to improve adherence and to identify the patients whose pharmacological pattern is poorly organized and who therefore are at higher risk of relapse. At the end of the group, our patients generally evaluate this round as a very interesting and useful exercise, and some of them comment that it changed the way they take their medication. It is appropriate to have the patients themselves advise each other as to how to take the medication because, since the therapists do not chronically take any medication, they cannot possibly achieve the modeling objective. Among the tricks, our patients discuss most frequently and among the most infrequent and strange ones, we can include the following:
  - Taking the medication at the same time with a daily routine act: some patients systematically take their medication when they brush their teeth or when they have breakfast and dinner.

- Using "pill reminder boxes" (special containers with the days of the week).
- Using some type of warning, such as the alarm of the clock.
- Using some reminder, such as changing the wristwatch.
- Writing down the taking of medication as an assignment to do in the daily planner, including with alarm if they have a palm pilot.
- Leaving medication blisters throughout the house or in different places (office, bag, bathroom).
- Writing "did you take your medication?" in the screensaver of the computer.
- Using the "traffic-light" technique, which consists of using a couple of round pieces of cardboard which are colored red on one side and green on the other. The patient starts the day with both cardboards on red placed in a visible location in the house; as he takes the medication, he turns the cardboards around. Thus, if at night before going to bed, he still finds a red cardboard, he will know that he did not take all the medication. This trick was infallible for one of our patients and, although it was not useful for the others, it inspired several versions with modifications which were helpful to the others.

- It is very important for each patient to find their own way of complying with the medication; however, the most compliant patients have is the intake of the medication so well integrated and rooted in their usual routine that very often they do not need to use any trick.
- The basic objective of this session is to make the patients associate poor adherence with relapses, and in order to achieve this association we must give as many examples as necessary. In general, it is the patients themselves who give these examples spontaneously.
- After reviewing the material, we give it to the patients together with the homework and we close the session.

## Useful tips

- For those patients who eventually "allow themselves" to start a hypomanic episode, we should let them know that only on very rare occasions does hypomania come by itself and in a limited episode, and almost always it predicts the inception of a depressive episode or the beginning of a manic or mixed picture; most patients understand the saying "the higher you go the harder the fall."

- It is very important to obtain that our patients do not associate hypomania or mania with virtuous or extremely fun periods, especially because many of them abandon the mood-stabilizing treatment seeking precisely this type of relapse, in other words because they have an "addictive" behavior toward mania. To avoid this situation it will be necessary to place special emphasis on the most unpleasant symptoms of these phases: anxiety, unrest, racing thoughts, or psychotic symptoms which the patients experience with a lot of suffering; thinking of these symptoms is usually a good reason to try to avoid a manic recurrence.

- It is very important to tackle the topic of side effects and teach the patients to distinguish between real side effects and the fear of future discomfort or problems and, in particular, make them learn to tolerate side effects that could be considered minor as compared to the magnitude of their bipolar disorder and the impact it has on their lives when it is decompensated.

- An issue that usually comes up in this session is the relationship between the social environment and psychotropic drugs, because in many cases the social circle or even the patient's family does not understand the need to take medication and sends messages such as "you are going to become stupid from so much medication," "one solves mental problems by oneself and not with pills", or "this medication is drugging you, you look like a zombie," which has a very negative impact on adherence. Just as one of the most important issues in the session of the first unit was "how do I tell (or should I tell) the others that I am bipolar," in this session it is important to tackle the topic of "how do I tell the others that I need to take medication chronically." Once again, we will insist that patients must select very carefully how and to whom they disclose such things. In general, we advise all patients to speak about their need for treatment with special emphasis on the more biological aspects of the disorder. On the other hand, there are cases in which certain intake is especially bothersome from a social viewpoint (e.g. intake at lunchtime if the patient has lunch at work), and this may cause constant forgetting and negligence and lead the patient to poor adherence. In these cases, it will be recommendable to advise patients to talk about this discomfort with their psychiatrist, since many times it is possible to group the doses in single intakes in the morning and at night, and avoid the opportunity to forget.

## Patient material

Approximately, half of the bipolar patients abandon their treatment during the first prescription year, and many others stop it in subsequent months. Practically, 7 of every 10 patients stop the medication at some time in their life, and 9 of every 10 bipolar patients think very seriously of abandoning it. Stopping the treatment, on the other hand, is the most common trigger of relapses.

The reasons that are most frequently argued to stop the medication are:

- Feeling bad because it is the medication and not the person controlling the mood.
- Believing that one is capable of controlling the bipolar disorder without need to take any drug.
- Missing hypomania.
- Denying the disorder.
- Overestimating the side effects.
- Being afraid of long-term consequences.
- Having erroneous beliefs about the medication ("it creates dependence," "it makes you stupid," etc.).
- Being misinformed.
- Lowering one's guard in periods of euthymia and not understanding the chronic character of the disorder.
- The beginning of a hypomanic or manic phase.

Lithium and, in general, stabilizers may avoid a relapse in most cases, but for this purpose it must be taken correctly, without omitting any intake. Using the tactic of taking lithium when one starts feeling poorly usually leads to a relapse, since it is a drug with very slow action. Taking mood stabilizers guarantees long periods of euthymia and these guarantee, in turn, a better quality of life.

The attitude of the family is crucial in maintaining therapeutic adherence, and for this attitude to be positive it will be essential for the patient's environment to be duly informed about the disorder and its treatment.

What are the risks of interrupting the treatment with lithium? Interrupting the treatment with lithium or any other mood stabilizer is associated with a sudden worsening of the natural evolution of the disorder and many times to hospitalization; more than half of the patients suffer a relapse in the

6 months after abandoning the mood stabilizer, and nine out of ten have a relapse during the following year. It has been observed that the risk of suicide increases spectacularly among the patients who have stopped taking their mood stabilizer. In addition, in the case of lithium, there is the added risk that the drug becomes inefficient when we start taking it again after having interrupted the treatment.

Certain patients argue that taking or not taking the medication makes no difference, because they have suffered relapses even while taking it. The possibility of suffering an episode never disappears, but the sure thing is that the probability of its occurring is much lower in medicated patients who, in addition, if they do have relapses, they will be shorter, less severe and of course more infrequent.

---

**Assignment 12**

Have you ever consumed alcohol, coffee, joints, cocaine, design drugs, acid, or other toxics? For what purpose? With what frequency are you consuming them currently? How do you believe they may affect your bipolar disorder?

---

# Avoiding substance abuse

Practically, half of bipolar patients, specifically 46%, meet DSM-IV (*Diagnostic and Statistical Manual for Mental Disorders 4th edition*) criteria of alcohol abuse or dependence. According to the data of the Epidemiologic Catchment Area (ECA), the risk for a bipolar patient to present with a drug dependence is more than six times higher than that of the population at large, and a little higher if we speak only of patients with type I bipolar disorder. One out of every three bipolar patients presents with a substance abuse problem as a comorbidity. On the other hand, many of our patients do not meet the criteria for substance abuse or dependence even though they consume alcohol or other substances with a certain assiduity, and we must take into account that the mere consumption of alcohol, cannabis and other toxics, even without reaching abuse quantities, can act as a trigger for new episodes.

Our program, far from claiming to be a specific program that tackles dual pathology, is designed to affect the consumption behavior more than the abuse or dependence, circumstances which would require a highly specialized program. In other words, the idea is to prevent substance consumption in order to control a potential triggering factor. To achieve this objective, we will not only dedicate the session to the substances traditionally considered toxic – alcohol, cannabis, cocaine and other stimulants, hallucinogens, opiates – but we will also dedicate considerable time to warn our patients about misuse of coffee, because many of them tend to drink it in excess and sometimes to use it as a stimulant to compensate their sub-threshold depressive symptomatology; this behavior obviously implies a risk, especially because of its impact on the quality of sleep. Most patients are not aware of this risk and attribute an excessive inter-individual variability to it ("the coffee does not affect me, because I continue sleeping correctly"). It is very important therefore to warn during the program not only about the risks of abuse, but also of the risks of incorrect consumption. General advice, for example, is that one must never drink coffee or beverages with caffeine after four in the afternoon, since it may affect our sleep up to 8 h after ingestion.

On the other hand, it is important to stress the four classic forms of interference between substance consumption and bipolar disorders, since this aspect may help our patients better understand their consumption problem:

1 Many patients start consuming toxics as a form of "self-medication," in other words seeking to alleviate some of their symptoms. They consume cocaine for their lack of energy or depressive apathy, and opiates, alcohol or cannabis for anxiety, etc. In this case we must warn our patients that the consumption of toxics worsens the evolution of the disorder.
2 The consumption of toxics is a powerful trigger of new episodes and, even though not all toxics have the same risk, it is essential to warn the patients on this point.
3 Furthermore, toxics may mask the affective symptoms and "pollute" their presentation, so that they may lead to confusion in diagnosis.
4 To convince the patients whose chronic consumption of small quantities of toxics does not induce new episodes, it is important to use the irrefutable argument of the worsening of the evolution of the disorder on the medium term.

The importance of avoiding toxic consumption to improve the evolution of the bipolar disorders is present throughout the program; in spite of the fact that we will only dedicate an *ad hoc* expression to this topic, it appears in many other sessions (causes and triggers, evolution, alternative treatments, course of action in case of decompensation, regularity, etc.).

# Psychoactive substances: risks in bipolar disorders

## Goal

Substance abuse or dependency problems are very frequent in the bipolar population, involving about 50% of patients according to some studies. Seven out of ten bipolar men abuse alcohol during mania, thus complicating its course. The goal of this session above all is for our patients to become aware of the risk, not of hard drugs (if indeed the distinction between hard and soft drugs makes any sense), but of more everyday-drugs like coffee and alcohol. This awareness is crucial because the number of bipolar patients who use caffeine is very high and the majority of them do not even view this behavior as a problem, although its effect on sleep and on comorbid pathologies that are very common in bipolar disorders such as panic attacks is very obvious.

## Procedure

- While the therapist talks informally to the group members, one of the co-therapists can write the following list on the blackboard:
  - Beer.
  - Wine.
  - Joints (marijuana).
  - Whisky, rum, and other hard liquors.
  - Acid ("trips").
  - Cocaine.
  - Amphetamines.
  - Stimulating beverages (Red Bull).
  - Cola drinks.

- – Coffee.
- – Ecstasy and other designer drugs.
- Once our informal chat is over, we put the following question openly to the whole group: "Which of the substances listed on the blackboard do you think are potential dangers for a person suffering from bipolar disorder?" Most of the patients will exclude some of the substances from the list, generally coffee and cola drinks but also sometimes wine and beer, and even marijuana. The basic message of this session is that all the items on the list are toxic substances with abuse and dependency potential, and accordingly inadvisable for a person suffering from bipolar disorder. It is essential to start by hitting hard with this message, although the nuances will be brought out later in the session.
- This message will probably give rise to an fervent debate among the patients, which we allow to proceed, only adding a few technical notes from our area of knowledge.
- The debate is usually confused because the patients tend to mix up data on the various toxic agents. A good way to present it is to divide the list into groups of different toxins. We usually start with alcoholic beverages and write "Alcoholic Beverages" in big letters on the blackboard, and announce that for 20 min we will debate their use and their problems in relation to bipolar disorder and its treatment (interaction with psychoactive drugs). It is desirable to divide up the time between the various agents according to their frequency of use and the polemic they generate:
  - – Alcohol: 20 min.
  - – Marijuana: 10 min.
  - – Cocaine, acid, and designer drugs: 10 min.
- This time distribution will of course vary according to the profile of our patient group. We have sometimes found that most of them are used to be habitual marijuana users, so it was necessary to spend almost the entire session on the myth that marijuana has no harmful effects on mental health; in other groups, however, none of the patients was a habitual marijuana user and it had the connotation of a risky substance. The same happens with alcohol, although this is generally the agent most widely consumed by our patients and the population at large.
- The discussion around coffee always has to be initiated by us, as most of our patients are unaware of the hazards of coffee in bipolar disorder. We

emphasize that it is no trivial thing, because coffee is a potential inducer of hypomania and anxiety, and because it is frequently abused in our patient population: it is by no means rare to find one or two patients in each of our psychoeducation groups who developed a clear dependency on caffeine, which was generally undiagnosed.

- As for smoking, we usually tackle this subject if there are smokers in the group, which is usually the case. In no event must we give the impression that, because smoking appears to have no significant effect on the course of bipolar disorder, we are encouraging our patients to carry on smoking. Obviously, we warn them of the risks involved in smoking for the physical health of any individual.
- We open the group up to a round of questions then after distributing the material and assignments, close the session.

## Useful tips

- The content of the session absolutely must not take on shades of "moral counseling," paternalistic warnings, or a police attitude. We explicitly tell our patients that we recommend avoiding marijuana, for example, for strictly medical reasons, remote from moral connotations.
- We can reinforce this position with various points:
  - Alcohol and coffee are perfectly legal but can be just as harmful as marijuana for a person suffering from bipolar disorder.
  - Doughnuts and cookies are legal, but a diabetic must not have them. Anchovies are legal as well as being very rich – but a hypertensive must not try them. For the same reasons, a person suffering bipolar disorder should not try marijuana, however much he may like it. There is no legalistic attitude in this advice, and we are not here to ban anything, just tell you what substances are dangerous for your disorder.
- Some of the usual questions from our patients during this session are directed at getting the psychologist to give them the permission they could not get from their psychiatrists about moderate consumption of particular agents, generally alcohol. So we have to be very cautious about answering questions such as "If I'm euthymic, can I drink a glass of wine if I go out to dinner?," "Can I drink half a glass of wine to toast someone?" or "Can I drink a shandy (beer and lemonade) from time to time?" Although

we could give this permission to some patients, it would dilute the general message of the session and would also involve a serious risk: during the psychoeducation group we cannot get to know our patients in the depth that their psychiatrist knows them so we are not in a position to evaluate the risk of alcohol abuse. The right answer to this kind of question in the group is "that's something you'll have to talk over with your psychiatrist," and of course we have to cut short advice from the rest of the group such as "I drank a stout of brandy every morning and nothing's happened to me yet," or "You have to know how to drink."

- Most of our patients react with skepticism to the news that coffee and cola drinks can trigger relapses in a bipolar patient, so that we often have to use one of the following strategies:
  - Explain to our patients the biological basis for the coffee-drinking risk in bipolar disorder (noradrenergic agonist).
  - Explain the physical problems associated with coffee abuse.
  - Explain in detail one case of decompensation due to coffee abuse suffered by one of our patients.

During the session, reinforce a report by any patient who has had problems because of coffee.

- In one of our groups it actually happened that one of the patients experienced decompensation, apparently after getting a new job, and stopped coming to group because he had to be hospitalized for a mixed episode. When he returned to group, he told everyone that his new job was a sales rep for a coffee company, so that he had to drop into bars all day and usually offered his coffee to the owner to try and convince him to change brands. As a result, he drank over 10 cups of coffee a day, which may have been a key factor in his decompensation. This anecdote was very useful for the patients in this particular group, and we also tell it to the other groups, pointing out that the abuse does not even have to be that high to bring about decompensation.

## Patient materials

By "drugs" we mean all substances, whether legal (alcohol, tobacco, coffee) or illegal (marijuana, cocaine, hallucinogens) that can modify the state of consciousness, behavior, thoughts, and emotions, and create dependency or abuse behaviors. Most studies available indicate that up to 60% of bipolar patients abuse or depend on some drug, especially alcohol. This abuse *obviously makes the course and prognosis of the disorder worse*. Patients who consume toxic agents experience more episodes and admissions than those who refrain from consuming them.

Many bipolar patients who have substance abuse or dependency problems enter into a self-medicating relationship with drugs, that is, they seek relief for some of their symptoms, generally before being diagnosed with bipolar disorders. Frequently, the alcohol abuse of many alcoholic bipolar patients began when the substance was used as an "anxiolytic," before proper treatment was received, or patients dependent on cocaine began their relationship with the drug hoping – consciously or unconsciously – that using it would cheer them up when they were in the apathy or depression phase. This type of behavior apart from generating dependency and an endless list of physical problems, consumption of toxic agents eventually worsens the psychiatric symptomatology:

- *Alcohol* causes depression in the medium term, increases anxiety, destructures sleep, reduces impulse control, causes cognitive deterioration, increases aggressiveness, and may cause the appearance of psychotic symptoms and mania.
- *Marijuana* creates an amotivational syndrome characterized by great apathy; it depresses, can trigger a mania, interfere with sleep, increase anxiety, and cause psychotic symptoms in the form of paranoid delirium.
- *Cocaine* all by itself can trigger any type of episode: rapid cycling, anxiety, aggressiveness, psychotic symptoms, interference with sleep, cognitive deterioration, and many other symptoms that generally end up with constant hospital admissions.
- *Hallucinogens* and designer drugs also involve a great deal of risk, even if they are taken just once, and may make hospitalization necessary. They bring on psychotic symptoms such as visual and/or auditory hallucinations and delirium in any individual, even a person without a mental disorder, and these symptoms can persist for a long time with flashbacks (repetition of the symptoms weeks or months after the substance was taken). In a person with bipolar disorder, taking hallucinogens or designer drugs can cause mania, psychotic symptoms, anxiety, etc.

The danger of *coffee* is mainly its ability to alter sleep structure. As we know, enjoying the right amount of high-quality sleep is essential for keeping bipolar disorders compensated. We emphasize sleep "quality." Many people say that even when they drink coffee after dinner they sleep 8 h; they may sleep 8 h, but their sleep is probably of poor quality. It is advisable not to drink coffee for 8 h before bedtime, as the half-life of coffee is just 8 h. On the other hand, there is absolutely no harm in having a couple of cups of coffee in the daytime (such as one in the morning and the other after lunch), although this depends on each individual because the effect of coffee is highly variable. During depressive phases, it is acceptable to drink a little more coffee, always in the morning and provided there is no anxiety. Coffee is totally inadvisable in anxious patients and patients with a history of panic attacks. Also, no type of caffeine (coffee or cola drinks) should be drunk during hypomanic, manic, and mixed phases, or with a suspicion that one of them is starting.

As far as *smoking* is concerned: there is no doubt that bipolar patients smoke more than the rest of the population, basically for two reasons: (a) to try to control the anxiety and (b) to try to alleviate some side effects of the drugs taken for mania, although this is not done intentionally. From the psychiatric standpoint, smoking does not involve serious risks, although we know it is very harmful to the physical health. In any event, the only problem with bipolar patients smoking is when they quit smoking. We have six important tips:

1  Never try to quit smoking during a decompensation.
2  It is advisable to attempt to quit smoking in periods of greatest stability (6 months euthymia or more).
3  Do not try to stop suddenly.
4  It is advisable to seek the help of psychological therapies to quit smoking in a rational, risk-free manner.
5  The use of substitutes is recommended (nicotine chewing gum or patch) to avoid the withdrawal syndrome, which may give rise to anxiety and irritability.
6  The use of quitting drugs such as bupropion is entirely contraindicated in bipolar patients, except during depressive phases – if prescribed by the psychiatrist – as bupropion is an antidepressant and can hence cause hypomanic or manic switch.

Another aspect that calls for comment is the misuse or abuse by some patients of their medications, which become treated like street drugs. The only psychoactive drugs that can create dependency if not used properly and strictly according to the doctor's prescription are the anxiolytics (benzodiazepines such as alprazolam, diazepam, or lorazepam). Thus, although the doctor should avoid prescribing these drugs to patients at risk of addiction, we must always remember the importance of following the psychiatrist's prescription to the letter.

---

**Assignment 13**

How do you believe you can detect hypomania or mania before it's too late? What behaviors can tell you that you are decompensating?

---

# Early detection of new episodes

Unit 4 is devoted to teaching patients how to identify a relapse, take prompt action from the behavioral standpoint, and work out an emergency drug treatment plan. Early detection of relapses is a technique that has already been discussed, especially in individual format, and many of our patients benefit from its being built into a group psychoeducation program.

Perhaps the best study on individual psychological intervention in bipolar disorders is the one by Perry et al. (1999); the type of intervention was a variable number of sessions, between 7 and 12, in which the therapist used a distinctly psychoeducative approach in helping patients to identify their most habitual relapse signals. The results indicate that the patients in the treatment group ($N = 34$) took longer to experience a manic relapse and, at the end of the follow-up period, had a smaller number of manic relapses than the control group ($N = 35$). It seems that there was no prevention effect for depressive episodes.

In our program we place special emphasis on early detection of hypomanic and manic symptoms for various reasons, most important of which are:

- The speed with which hypomania warning signs ("prodromes") become a full-blown episode is far greater than in the case of depression. While in depression several weeks usually elapse between the first warning signs and the actual episode, in the case of hypomania and manic this can happen in a matter of days or hours.
- We have (almost)-immediate-acting drugs to stop the start of a manic episode, while this is not true for depression.
- Many patients have serious difficulty in identifying hypomania, while the suffering that usually accompanies depression acts as an alarm signal. However, this is not true for all bipolar patients, many of whom have

depression without sadness, characterized mainly by fatigue, inhibition, and apathy, sometimes with little suffering or desperation.
- Many patients tend to "give themselves permission" to live through their initial hypomanic signs without taking any action to abort the episode, and this happens because very often the patient has a near-addictive relationship with mania. This is why any action identifying the early signs of hypomania as something pathological and a cause for concern by the patient is especially important.

Nevertheless, we do also devote one group session to identifying depressive episodes. Our approach to identifying early signs consists of three steps: of these, the first and second are generally worked during the group program, while the third step usually requires individual intervention, although this is not essential in all cases.

## Step 1: Information – frequent relapse signals

- The goal is a didactic one, namely to teach the patients what are the commonest warning signs of both depression and (hypo)mania.
- This is done in group, generally in the corresponding session (Session 15 for (hypo)mania and Session 16 for depression, see pp. 163 and 169), although it is also possible to deal with the subject in Sessions 4 and 5, corresponding to the symptoms (see pp. 78 and 85). In the latter case, once we have made up a list of symptoms as a group, we ask our patients to tell us which ones they feel could function as alarm signals if present in a mild form.
- The first exercise in Step 1 consists of making up a list of alarm signals of a particular type of episode, which we compile by going around the group for comments, which are written on the blackboard. If we believe the group is not yet up to the task, we offer a list of symptoms instead of a list of signals, then ask the patients to choose which symptoms could act as relapse signals.
- We then discuss with the group the warning signs we consider doubtful. As always, it is best to facilitate and let the group do the discussing.
- Once we have the definitive list, we go on to Step 2, asking the patients to choose which of the common relapse signals are not useful for their particular case, and to make an individual list of those that are useful. Normally, we ask our patients to prepare this list at home, and we go over it at the next session.

## Step 2: Individualization – identification of one's own warnings or operational warnings

- The goal of this step is to individualize, that is adapt the information from Step 1 to everyone's particular case. We try to have the patients to identify which warning signs appear regularly in each type of episode.
- To make Step 2 accessible and workable for our patients, we have to incorporate the figure of the "ally": each patient must appoint one or more "ally": a trusted person or persons who can help with early identification of an episode and rapid intervention. An "ally" or support person must have the following characteristics:
  - Have sufficient knowledge about bipolar disorders.
  - Have practically daily contact with the patient. In cases where personal contact is not possible, telephone contact is acceptable.
  - Have no conflictive relationship with the patient, so that the symptoms could be used as a "weapon" or misused in some other way. In certain families it is not advisable for the parents to be the support people for their bipolar child, as they could mismanage the advice about sleep and use this in generational arguments. We have also seen cases of spouses who, during an argument, accuse our patients of being irritable even though they really are not. In any event, in most cases the support person will be the parent, sibling, or spouse of our patient.
- It is advisable for the patient, with the help of the support person, to work at home on making a list of warning signs that are useful to him or her.
- It is important for the list to contain not only the warning sign but also an operational definition of it or an example.
- Each patient must decide what warning signs are useful for him or her, depending on their temperament, personality, circumstances, and surroundings.
- It is important to teach the patient that characteristics can become warning signs.
- A valid warning sign must:
  - *Be regular for all episodes*: This means that it must clearly and always repeat in all episodes of the same type.
  - *Be easily identifiable*: We cannot choose warning signs that the patient has difficulty in clearly identifying (e.g. racing thoughts which, although

they occur regularly in many of our patients when a hypomania episode starts are not ideal as a warning sign because most patients do not identify them easily, at least in the first stages). We strongly encourage to select behaviors as warning signs, and avoid selecting thoughts or emotions.

- *Not lead to arguments*: We exclude as valid warning signs any that could lead to arguments between the patient and the ally. For example, irritability is not useful for some patients because the argument about the warning sign can "cause" it to appear.
- *Escalate to the symptom*: Warning signs that do not present until the episode is already advanced are not useful, nor are those that indicate that the episode may appear full blown in only a few hours time.

## Step 3: Specialization – prodromes of prodromes, or early warning signs

- As the name suggests, in this step the patient claims "specialization" in their own case, beyond knowledge of their own relapse signs. The point is to identify the signals that precede the warning signs – "warnings of warnings."
- This type of early warning usually consists of a behavioral or cognitive change, or a qualitatively different perception. It is usually personal to each individual and rarely repeats in two different patients. These are not changes that are pathological *per se*, as they would not be an alarm in another patient, yet they are pathognomonic for an individual patient.
- Early warning signals can be of various types:
  - *Symptom warning*: The subtle appearance of a behavioral change that in time may give rise to a warning sign or a symptom. Some patients tend to change their wardrobe a great deal during manic phases, so a subtle change in dress can be a warning sign (for one of our patients, a truly pathognomonic sign of mania was starting to wear sunglasses).
  - *Perceptual changes*: These changes are not changes in sensory perception, which would obviously be an actual symptom, but discrete changes in, for example, how colors are seen (generally perceived as brighter at the start of hypomania). This type of warning sign is tremendously reliable in the case of some patients; one of them, for example, "turns on the alarm light" when he starts to dwell too long on the reflections of lighted signs (traffic lights, neon signs outside the stores, etc.) which normally go unnoticed.

– *Behavioral changes not associated with symptoms*: Although infrequent, or at least difficult to detect, these changes are almost always predictive, and may be changes in behavior with no apparent symptomatic value that are repeatedly associated with the start of an episode. Some patients, for example, change their cigarette brand, the way they answer the phone, the newspaper they usually buy, the position they like to play when playing fusball or the route they take to work. Changes in some customary favorites (music, books, or even food) are also very significant.

One very useful way of working is to use lists. At each step, whether individually or in group, we can ask the patient to make out a list. Specifically, these are the lists with which we generally work:

1  *General list of symptoms*: This is created in Sessions 4 and 5 (see pp. 78 and 85) with a basically informational objective. We try to give an exhaustive list containing both the appropriate medical terminology and the colloquial terminology used by the patients to name each symptom. In the first phases of treatment, when our patients still have not learned the medical terminology, many of them use this list like a dictionary. We should add here that we have to advise our patients during their visits always to report their behavioral, cognitive, or mood changes just as they happen, without using medical nomenclature, as very often the patient can over-interpret or underinterpret a symptom, thus confusing the professional.

2  *General list of warning signs*: This corresponds to Step 1 of this fourth unit (see p. 157). Normally, it is created jointly by the members of the group during Sessions 15 and 16 (see pp. 163 and 169). The therapist must make sure the patients do not just repeat the list of symptoms, but cross out the ones that do not serve as warnings. In some groups it is very useful to start the list by writing *General Symptom List* on the blackboard then crossing out those that do not have a clear and possible warning utility.

3  *Personal list of operational warning signs*. Usually, the *General Warnings List* is used as a starting point; the patient follows the steps described below with the help of the support person at home and the consulting therapist, or in the corresponding psychoeducation session:

   (a) Assign each warning sign on the list to categories: "present at all starts of a phase," "frequent," "occasional," "rarely present," or "never present." Cross out the signs that *never* occur with this patient, and keep the rest.

(b) Assign an operational definition to each general sign kept on the list, a definition that has to be valid for the individual patient. For example, if the warning sign in the *General Warnings List* is "increased physical exercise," the operational definition for an individual patient could be "start bicycling to school" provided this behavior is clearly non-routine, that is if the patient definitely does not go to school by bicycle unless he is starting an episode.

(c) Score each operational sign according to how easy it is to identify (4: very easily identifiable, 3: identifiable, 2: difficult to identify, and 1: practically impossible to identify).

(d) Reorganize the classification of general warning signs by frequency, and also give them a score (4: present at all phase starts, 3: frequent, 2: occasional, and 1: rarely present).

(e) Add the scores given in steps 3 and 4 and arrange the list from the highest to the lowest score. To be functional, it is advisable for the final list of operational signs to have 5 to 10 items; if the patient's final list exceeds this number, the lowest-scoring items should be crossed out.

4  *List of early warning signs:* Very often, when making up the *Personal List of Operational Warnings* of the patient narrates and describes behavioral or cognitive changes that are difficult to classify as symptoms but are very indicative (and sometimes pathognomonic) of the start of decompensation. The list of early or advance warning signals should be prepared in the context of an individual visit, rarely during the psychoeducation group, although in some cases clear early/advance signs may appear during the psychoeducation sessions, in which case the therapist should reinforce them. The early signs are generally very concrete and easily describable behaviors (the patient starts to smoke, listens to a different kind of music from usual, has a very specific physical sensation; we note here the case of a patient who explained that he felt his blood was "effervescing" before beginning a hypomanic phase, and another patient who felt his "head was hot" when he started to become depressed). Participation of the support person ("ally") may facilitate preparation of the list of early signs in the case of very obvious behavioral changes, but it is generally a good idea for the final list to depend exclusively on the patient. The early signs are added to the list of operational signs in making up the final list of signs.

## How to use the list of signs?

Once the patient has made up a list of about 10 items for hypomania/mania, another for depression, and in some cases where especially necessary, a third for mixed episodes (that may be a combination of the list for depression and the one for mania), we have to work out with the patient (and if he agrees, the support person as well) how to use this list. Generally, the patient is advised to use the lists daily. Many patients set up a document in their personal computer and use it as an everyday reminder, others include it in their personal date book, and others in their electronic calendar; whichever way it is used, the following criteria must always be followed:

- If, after reviewing the list, you match one or none of the items, do not do anything to change behavior.
- If you match two items for 3 days in a row, you should consult with your support person.
- If you match three or more items in a single day, it is time to put an emergency plan into effect.

# Early detection of *mania and hypomanic episodes*

## Goal

The goal of this session is for patients to learn to detect their (hypo)manic relapses in time, and make their own lists of operational early signs so that these are available for identification of future episodes.

## Procedure

- The session can begin with a reminder of the symptoms of mania and hypomania, and the difference between the two as, although this may seem strange, at this stage in the program there are still patients who do not have the clear distinction between depression and mania.
- To meet our objective, we quickly go around the group to name all the symptoms of mania.
- We ask the group the following questions: "Do you believe all these symptoms can act as alarm signals? Which should we remove from the list? Should we add anything?"
- The answers to these questions will lead to some important considerations for the session: some symptoms appear so suddenly that they are of no use as warning signs, while other – non-pathological – behaviors are actually good indicators of a relapse.
- With the co-operation of the group, we go around again to come up with the *General Warnings List*.
- We explain to the patients how to prepare the *Personal List of Operational Warnings*, always emphasize the need to individualize the knowledge of the disorder: I am trying to learn not about *the* illness of bipolar disorder but about *my* bipolar disorder – an idea that perfectly fits the concept the patients have of their psychiatric disorder.

- Another important point in this session is the "ally" or support person. One of the homework assignments will be to find the proper support person for detecting relapses (of all types) and to prepare an emergency plan. This point may generate debate among the patients but, following the guidelines noted at the start of Unit 4 (see p. 156), deciding on the support person is obviously the individual responsibility of each patient.
- We distribute the materials and homework, and end the session.

## Useful tips

- One useful comparison to help the patients understand the need for early detection and treatment of (hypo)mania is the avalanche: a manic episode works like an avalanche. At the beginning, it is just a little snowball sliding smoothly down the slope, not apparently dangerous, and you could stop it with your hand. As it rolls down the side of the mountain, however, there comes a point where it cannot be stopped without heroic measures, and it may do a great deal of damage.
- A warning sign is not a symptom, and the difference between the two terms is essential if the patients are to utilize the content of this session. To make this difference clear, we may draw the "mountain picture" (Figure 7): we draw a parabola (i.e. a mountain) on the blackboard to present mania. We explain that we are not interested in detecting the symptoms at the top of the mountain, when it is generally too late for any preventive action and the only possible intervention is prescribing high-dose antimanic drugs and even, sometimes, hospitalization; rather we want to detect them at the beginning of the slope. We can ask the group to situate each symptom and each sign at one point on the mountain, depending on when it appears. With this exercise we stress the distinction between valid signals and symptoms.
- The behavioral and cognitive changes occurring in the (hypo)manic episodes can be divided into:
  - (a) *Quantitative* changes in which a normal function is generally observed to increase (racing speech, racing thoughts, increased activity, or energy) or diminish (decreased need for sleep) and
  - (b) *Qualitative* changes, meaning that a new behavior or cognition appears in the patient's recent life (irritability and discussions in people who are not usually irritable, new interests, start taking toxic substances, etc.).

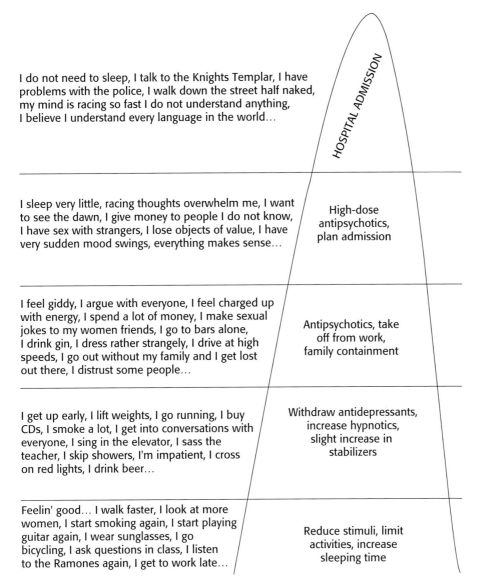

I do not need to sleep, I talk to the Knights Templar, I have problems with the police, I walk down the street half naked, my mind is racing so fast I do not understand anything, I believe I understand every language in the world…

*HOSPITAL ADMISSION*

I sleep very little, racing thoughts overwhelm me, I want to see the dawn, I give money to people I do not know, I have sex with strangers, I lose objects of value, I have very sudden mood swings, everything makes sense…

High-dose antipsychotics, plan admission

I feel giddy, I argue with everyone, I feel charged up with energy, I spend a lot of money, I make sexual jokes to my women friends, I go to bars alone, I drink gin, I dress rather strangely, I drive at high speeds, I go out without my family and I get lost out there, I distrust some people…

Antipsychotics, take off from work, family containment

I get up early, I lift weights, I go running, I buy CDs, I smoke a lot, I get into conversations with everyone, I sing in the elevator, I sass the teacher, I skip showers, I'm impatient, I cross on red lights, I drink beer…

Withdraw antidepressants, increase hypnotics, slight increase in stabilizers

Feelin' good… I walk faster, I look at more women, I start smoking again, I start playing guitar again, I wear sunglasses, I go bicycling, I ask questions in class, I listen to the Ramones again, I get to work late…

Reduce stimuli, limit activities, increase sleeping time

Figure 7 Example of a "mountain of symptoms," with corresponding therapeutic interventions.

As warning signs, the qualitative changes are much more useful as they tend not to cause confusion or arguments. In the case of quantitative changes, the patient can have problems in knowing how much thinking or talking speed is indicative of a relapse, or how much optimism should be considered too much (this is logical, by the way). These doubts can lead to an episode not being identified until it is too late for early intervention. The only quantitative change that we could consider valid would be the reduction in sleeping hours, as this is easily operational: two nights sleeping less than 6 or 7 h would be enough to switch on the alarm in most patients.

## Patient material

Detecting a relapse in time is crucial for avoiding it. As soon as the patient detects the first signs of a relapse, it is probably less intense, less disruptive, and the amount of medication needed to treat it is less. Detecting relapse signals (what we can call "warnings") early is a process that requires both the persons suffering from bipolar disorder and the people around them (family, spouse, or friends) to learn to recognize small changes in behavior. These changes are often crucial in identifying a relapse and can initiate rapid, effective intervention.

We are all used to suspecting we are starting a flu if we detect signs at bedtime such as excessive fatigue, runny nose, physical malaise, temperature changes, or sneezing. These alarm signals send us to the appropriate "emergency plan": we start taking medication and postpone the next day's commitments. A bipolar patient should be able to carry out the same process with their disorder, that is, be able to detect the signs early and start an emergency plan.

There are certain changes in behavior and thinking that usually indicate the start of hypomanic decompensation in most cases. The most common are:

- Fewer hours sleeping.
- Feeling of "lost time" about the hours spent asleep.
- Impatience.
- Irritability or increased number of arguments.

- Higher energy level.
- Appearance of new interests or recovery of interests from former stages of life (e.g. listening to music one used to listen some 15 years ago).
- Talking faster, so that the people around us notice.
- Driving faster.
- Appearance of new projects.
- Increased sexual desire, so that the patient often becomes more attracted than usual to persons of the opposite sex (or the same sex in the case of homosexuals).
- Changing the style of dress.

In any event, since everyone is different and each patient is a world unto themself, not all these signs will serve in all cases and without a doubt some of them will be more useful than others. So everyone needs to write their own list and adapt it to their own personality, if necessary with the aid of someone they are close to. In some cases, certain signals such as talking very fast will not be useful if the patient talks fast *habitually*; rather, certain other signals will be far more indicative of decompensation. Trying to write one's own list of alarm signals with the help of a trusted person if necessary is thus a very interesting exercise. This exercise lets us get to know ourselves better, and define clearly what signals should start to concern us by indicating a relapse into hypomania or mania.

Coming around a circle of group members, we can try to find relapse signals that are apparently meaningless but repeat episode after episode and are practically personal and not transferable to others (e.g. starting or stopping smoking, starting doing physical exercise, changing the type of reading, having a particularly physical sensation, etc.) This type of signal will be especially useful for detecting a new episode, so it is very interesting to try and find them.

The process of symptom monitoring described is, of course, a learning process and we have to bear in mind:

- Our personality prior to decompensation.
- The symptoms that occurred in prior episodes.
- How the symptoms would vary with each episode.
- What triggers usually affect us and cause the appearance of a new episode.
- Where is the limit at which it is important to take action.

Learning the life-chart technique, which we explained in previous sessions (see p. 101), can also help us detect possible triggers and relapse signals as on occasion these are constant.

How do we know whether a mood fluctuation is normal or if we should be alarmed? Obviously, everyone spontaneously experiences mild mood fluctuations that are entirely normal (whether we are bipolar or not); some day we all get out of bed on the wrong side and we all experience mood fluctuations in reaction to external factors (worries, good or bad news), stress, illness, fatigue, hormonal changes, etc. In the case of people who suffer from bipolar disorder, there is also the possibility that these fluctuations are due to initial decompensation of the disorder, and sometimes it can be difficult to distinguish these fluctuations from others.

The basic difference between normal mood swings and those specific to the disorder is that the former, whether or not they are caused by outside events, tend to disappear after a few hours, while those associated with the disorder tend to become worse as time passes. As intense as the joy associated with good news may be, it abates slowly as the hours go by, just as the impact of bad news will dwindle after a few hours or days.

Mood by itself does not give us much information about a decompensation, so that it is useful to look for other signals less associated with mood (sleep changes, irritability, changes in activities, etc.). In any event, it is very difficult to state that one is suffering a relapse if only one aspect has changed, and it is better to look for other items that have changed too. For example, we are all "entitled" to feel irritable from time to time, or be more optimistic or more impatient, or have greater sexual desire, without this being an alarm signal. However, if a couple of these changes occur simultaneously, we can start to ask whether this is a normal change.

---

**Assignment 14**

Draw up your own *List of Operational Warnings* (must contain at least seven items).

---

**Assignment 15**

How do you believe you can detect depression before it is too late? What behaviors can tell you decompensation is happening?

## Session 16

# Early detection of *depressive and mixed episodes*

## Goal

The goal of this session is to teach patients to detect their depressive episodes as soon as possible; this is not as easy as it sounds because many of them have difficulty in detecting the first signs, especially in the case of inhibited or anergic depressions with a low cognitive load and little mental suffering. Sometimes patients do not see a doctor until they have been seriously depressed for several weeks.

## Procedure

- After an informal conversation and answering the patients' questions, we can spend the first half hour of this session going over the first assignment we gave last session to see how many patients have been able to drawing up their own *Personal List of Operational Warnings* and their *List of Early Warning Signs*, which the group and the therapist can help to improve.
- The next step can be to go round the group and list symptoms of depression on the blackboard.
- Just as we did in Session 15 (see p. 163), with the aid of the group we can cross out some symptoms that are not useful as warning signs, and explain clearly why we are doing so.
- We go round the group again to write the *General List of Warning Signs*.
- Finally, we try to identify three or four operational signs for each patient. In the majority of groups we have run so far, it is not too difficult to bring our patients to this point with respect to depressive episodes, and sometimes early signs have even been found.

- If necessary, we go over the material prepared for the session, where various signs are cited explicitly. We rarely have to go back to it, as the majority of warning signs appear during the session and are fully discussed.
- We distribute the materials and assignments, and close the session.

## Useful tips

- It may be that talking about depression or its warning signs is not comfortable for some of our patients, so that humor may be used to lighten up provided this is done with the greatest respect and fits our therapeutic style.
- The concept of "depression without sadness" may be new to many patients and it should be explained in detail wherever possible, perhaps with the help of a member of the group who has suffered this type of depression.
- If we talk about memory and attention problems as possible early signs, we have to spend time discussing the cognitive dysfunctions in bipolar disorders – those associated with a certain episode, those that are drug related, and those that are permanent.
- Probably many patients will vociferously recount their bad experiences with family members who interfered or did not understand the disorder. As always, this is somewhat hot-tempered reaction must not be countered, as it is usually very authentic, but the positive point must be made that there are psychoeducation groups for families of bipolar patients (if there are such groups in the center) and informative books on the issue. We can also suggest visits by family members with the psychiatrist to receive information.

## Patient material

Although identifying depression is not as urgent as identifying a manic phase, and although the suffering associated with the beginning of a depression may alert us the start of a depressive phase, which clearly does not happen with mania or hypomania, it is still important to learn to identify the warning signs that may indicate the beginning of a depression.

As we have said, the majority of patients usually have no difficulty in identifying a depression, as the *psychic suffering* (sadness, anxiety, feelings of inadequacy, fatigue) acts as a messenger. To be sure, someone who is starting to undergo this kind of suffering wants to avoid it at all costs and, if properly informed that it is an illness, will seek help from a psychiatrist and psychologist. There are two exceptions:

1  The person is suffering but does not know or realize that this suffering is associated with the start of a depressive phase, so that he seeks help far away from health professionals and in some cases may consume alcohol or other drugs to cheer up. Many bipolar patients start a substance dependency or abuse problem for this reason, without being aware that substances like alcohol or cocaine make the depressive symptoms worse in the medium term, just by themselves.

2  In bipolar disorder we frequently encounter *depression without sadness* characterized mainly by fatigue, physical discomforts, increased hours of sleep, and inner void. Sometimes none of these symptoms makes the patient suspect he is depressed, but he thinks he has some type of non-psychiatric pathology (many believe they have anemia or fear cancer or progressive dementia) and consults doctors who are not psychiatrists.

On the other hand, we have to differentiate between the intervention necessary if the start of a manic picture is identified (quickly make a psychiatry appointment, increase the dose of some drugs) and the proper action when a depressive episode is detected. Although some patients agree with their psychiatrist on the possibility of increasing the dose of antimania or hypnotic drugs when they detect a sign of hypomania, mania, or mixed state, this action (altering the dose of a drug) is inappropriate in the case of depression: the patient *should never start to take antidepressants or increase their dosage without consulting the psychiatrist*. The first step, once the psychiatrist or psychologist is contacted, is to make behavioral changes to see that the activity pattern changes as little as possible, even if this takes extra effort. Suddenly taking antidepressants may start sudden switch into mania or rapid cycling, both of which only complicate the course of the disorder.

One of the most frequent signs of depression is *apathy*, involving a deteriorated activity pattern and neglect of some important tasks. This neglect, in its turn, brings on reproaches from others and oneself, which can erode self-esteem, aggravate the depressive symptoms, and cause the start of a self-sustaining depression spiral.

A drop in academic and job performance is also frequent, as are memory and attention problems, which are sometimes the first signs of the episode.

*Fatigue* and physical malaise are also very characteristic signs, and if the patient does not detect them properly they may give rise to symptoms.

A very valuable sign for the majority of patients is loss of interest in activities that were usually pleasant, or *enjoying them less*, without arriving at the classical anhedonia of depression. For example, the patient goes to the movies but does not appreciate them as much, does not enjoy playing soccer with friends, or is not interested in their conversations (whereas he was before). One very useful alarm signal, especially in young patients, is for two weekends to go by in which they prefer to stay at home rather than go out with friends.

Starting to worry about matters that were not worries before, or going over and over things in one's head, are also alarm signals. For some people, talking less or not knowing what to say can be a good indicator.

Sadness, which is the best-known depression symptom, is not a good indicator because patients usually attribute it to some past or present event (if you think about it, there is always some good reason for being sad, just as there is always some good reason for feeling happy).

The comments of those trusted by the patient may be useful in detecting a new depressive episode, provided these people are properly informed about bipolar disorder; on the other hand they can misinterpret the first signs of depression as signs of withdrawing or laziness, and contribute even more to the depression by undermining the patient's self-esteem.

---

**Assignment 16**

Make up your own *List of Operational Warning Signs* for depression.

---

**Assignment 17**

Once a decompensation is detected, what should you do? What are the appropriate actions for the start of a depression or hypomania?

# Session 17

# What to do when a *new phase* is detected?

## Goal

The goal of this session is to provide the patients in the group with a structured action plan if any decompensation begins. It is not a session designed to improve any symptoms by cognitive–behavioral intervention as, let us point out one more time, patients in psychoeducation must be euthymic. The goal of the session is prevention, that is, for our patients to learn techniques or acquire resources while they are euthymic that can later serve them during a decompensation.

## Procedure

- In a single session we will discuss how to act with all types of decompensation. It is advisable not to mix up useful tips for mixed episodes, hypomania, and mania – which are practically the same – with tips for depression, as this may confuse our patients. Thus, we have to divide the session time in the most appropriate way according to our patient profile, and reinforce this or that point according to explicit requests from the group members. Our experience tells us that it is usually necessary to spend more time on mixed episodes, hypomania, and mania than depression. We will now relate the content of a session with 50 min spent on mixed episodes, hypomania, and mania and 30 min on depression, leaving you, the reader, to allocate the time in your own future groups.
- Before going into appropriate action at the start of a decompensation, we have to know what resources our patients have available for a mixed or (hypo)manic decompensation, so we can reinforce the right ones and advise against the wrong ones. It is useful to go around the group and write the replies on the blackboard.

- We give the patients some time for debate and discussion among themselves of the best methods; we then talk about the "ten commandments" in the session material.
- In relation to the points discussed, it is useful to give a number of examples of how to limit activities and prioritize the really important ones.
- Another important point is physical exercise: we usually talk about physical exercise as a natural antidepressant, highly indicated in euthymic periods and depression, or when depression is suspected, but completely inadvisable for mixed states and (hypo)mania or if this type of episode is suspected. Many patients become quite disconcerted when a health professional advises them not to do physical exercise at some stage in their life, especially after the media campaign (even using some trusted and well-known health professionals such as Jane Fonda or Arnold Schwarszenneger) touting the benefits of sports. We have to make this point especially clear to our patients and tell them that physical exercise is a stimulant, and any stimulant is ill advised if a mixed relapse or (hypo)mania is suspected.
- We go around the group asking for possible resources for depression in the same way as for mixed or (hypo)manic decompensation.
- We talk about each point in the "ten commandments" if there is a suspicion of depression.
- When they are euthymic, the patients are usually very creative and supply many ideas about what activities they can do to avoid depression, so it is important to foster discussion on this issue.
- We distribute the materials and assignments and close the session.

## Useful tips

- The idea of self-medication with small doses of antipsychotics as an emergency resource with impending mixed or (hypo)manic decompensation is controversial, even among health professionals. In any event, antipsychotics must be prescribed by a psychiatrist at an individual appointment with the patient, never in a psychoeducation group, as to a large degree their success depends on patients' skills: their ability to identify decompensations correctly, and know what type they are; their response to antipsychotics, whether there is a history of substance abuse (albeit infrequently, cases of antipsychotic abuse have been described and in fact one of our patients started to take more olanzapine doses for no apparent reason, that is without a preventive intention), and their relationship with the psychiatrist. So this is not an advice to be generalized to all cases, but we have very good experience with some patients that, with a suspected relapse, increase the clonazepam dose to normalize sleep or slightly increase the antipsychotic dose during a couple of days. We believe this is one of the most powerful action mechanisms of psychoeducation: not only improving adherence, but also making the guidelines flexible so that they can be adjusted to manage symptoms. This may explain why our patients with higher cognitive level may respond better to psychoeducation as they are the ones able to put it into practice. One of our patients, a university teacher whose cognitive function has been fully retained, has a very clear warning sign: changing her usual lectures to esoteric lectures. This sign usually appears 4–5 days before a decompensation, with no other warning signal or accompanying symptom. She has learned to take 15 drops of haloperidol for 2 days whenever she detects this sign (the anecdote goes 9 years back when atypical antipsychotics were still not an established treatment for mania; also, the drop presentation allows the medication to be precisely controlled). With this procedure, she went from one admission a year, which had been happening over the previous 3 years, to no admissions in subsequent years. This went on until on one occasion, 4 years later, she decided that she had been overusing haloperidol and decided to change tactics. This landed her in the hospital for several days; during those days the patient was able to read some Louise Haye but probably ended up regretting it.

- We never advise a patient to change the drug prescription if a depressive episode is suspected. Many patients have a degree of addiction to their elation stages and may abuse antidepressants if the psychiatrist opens the door to this possibility, small though it may be. Other patients habitually hover around the border of subsyndromic depression; they might misinterpret this fluctuation and start using antidepressants.
- To prepare an emergency plan, it is very useful for the patient to have contact telephone numbers handy for their psychiatrist and psychologist. We can give our patients what we call a "fire extinguisher card" (so dubbed by one of our patients) bearing the center telephone number, the name and

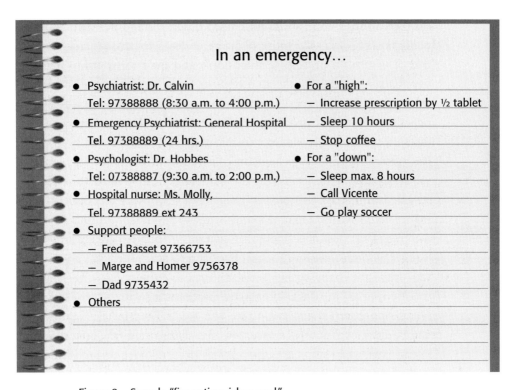

Figure 8    Sample "fire extinguisher card."

telephone number of their psychiatrist or other psychiatrists who could
step in, the psychologist, the team nurse, the center hours, and an emergency telephone number.

· We can complete the "fire extinguisher card" with three basic pieces of
advice for each case (Figure 8).

## Patient material

In the last few sessions we have learned to detect the start of a phase before
it is too late, but this would be no good if we did not know how to react to
this relapse. In this session we go back over some tips that, together with the
advice of the psychiatrist, may be very useful for nipping a relapse in the
bud. These are summarized in Chart 2.

**Chart 2.     What to do in a decompensation**

What to do for a hypomanic, mixed, or manic phase

1  If your *List of Operational Warnings* tells you that you may be relapsing, or if your support person suggests this possibility, the first step is to locate your psychiatrist or psychologist, even if by telephone, so that he or she can evaluate the relapse or tell you it is a non-pathological fluctuation.

2  Increase the number of sleeping hours to a minimum of 10, even if you need the drugs the psychiatrist prescribed for the emergency plan. Often, sleeping long hours for 3 or 4 days will be enough to head off a decompensation if detected in time.

3  Limit the number of activities and eliminate all that are not absolutely essential. Normally, the help of your ally will be needed to decide which activities are not essential. Remember: the only truly important thing is your health and avoiding relapses; this outweighs any job or social commitment.

4  Spend a maximum of 6 h being active. The rest of the day should be for resting or for relaxing, non-stimulating activities. You should behave as if you had the flu: lots of bed rest, a little TV, few outings, and lots of tranquility.

5  Never try to overcome your hyperactivity and increased energy by trying to exhaust yourself, doing lots of physical exercise to tire yourself out and so get back to normal. This is like trying to put out a fire with gasoline: the most activity you do, the more stimulated you will be, and the worse the episode will get. Physical exercise must be minimized.

6  Reduce stimuli: avoid exposure to highly stimulating environments (a discotheque, a demonstration, or a shopping center) and surround yourself with a relaxing environment (quiet, little light, few people).

7  Avoid stimulating beverages such as coffee, tea, cola drinks, and so-called energy drinks (containing taurine, ginseng, caffeine, or derivatives of these substances). Also avoid multivitamins because they sometimes contain some of these substances. Obviously, alcohol and other drugs should be avoided. Even if the psychiatrist has allowed you a small amount of alcohol, for example a beer at weekends, it is desirable not to drink if you suspect that you are starting an episode.

8  Limit spending: remove access to credit cards (someone you trust can hold on to them until the threatened episode disappears) and postpone all purchases for at least 48 h.

9 Never make important decisions if you suspect you are starting to suffer symptoms of hypomania. Until the psychiatrist or psychologist rules out the existence of an episode, you should postpone all decision-making.

10 Never give yourself permission to "go up a little more." Remember that the higher you go, the harder you will fall.

### What to do for a possible depressive phase

1 Try to reach your psychiatrist by phone. When a depressive phase starts, or when you suspect this is happening, you should not change psychiatrists, as the psychiatrist on duty may overevaluate your depressive symptoms without knowing that you have bipolar disorder, and this may lead to over-use of antidepressants.

2 You should never self-medicate for depressive symptoms. Carry on taking the medication prescribed by the psychiatrist.

3 Sleep 8h at most, as sleeping longer can worsen the depression. To limit sleeping time, it may be useful to schedule activities for the morning. Never sleep during siesta time.

4 Try to increase your activity level, even though this is just the opposite of what you want to do. Do not leave out any of your daily activities.

5 It is very important for you to do physical exercise; if you cannot go to the gym or go swimming, try to walk at least half an hour every day.

6 Do not make important decisions – these should be made only when you are fully lucid. They should not be influenced by the pessimism and despair characteristic of depressive states. If you make decisions at the beginning of a depression, the decision is probably being made by the depression, not by you.

7 Do not consume alcohol, marijuana, or cocaine to try to cheer yourself up or be more active: these substances will leave you even more depressed after a few hours. If you do not have anxiety problems, you can drink a couple of cups of coffee, in the morning, for stimulation.

8 Try to put notions of inferiority and pessimism in perspective: they are just the result of biochemical changes in the brain. If you talk about them to a trusted person or your "ally," they will probably tell you that you are blowing up the importance of these notions.

9 Try to keep to a regular schedule; many depressed people feel better in the afternoon, so they go to bed later and later, and end up with upside-down sleeping hours. It is best to go on living during the day and sleeping at night.

10 Move up your visit to the psychologist; he will give you advice on how to deal with this initial decompensation. If you have suicidal ideas, always talk about them.

---

**Assignment 18**

Draw up your own emergency plan and your "fire extinguisher card."

---

**Assignment 19**

What do you think is the importance of sleep in your disorder? Keep a record of how many hours you sleep, with your energy level and how you feel.

# Regular habits and stress management

Regular habits and stress management are extremely important in bipolar disorder, and belong in any complete treatment program. These two points are crucial for other psychological interventions (essentially interpersonal therapy and cognitive–behavioral therapy) and become the central axis of the theoretical and practical approach of these interventions, especially of interpersonal social-rhythm therapy. In our program, regular habit and stress management are presented from the earliest sessions as essential factors in keeping the disorder compensated and, like substance use, are part of almost every session. This is why we decided to handle these points in greater depth in two sessions, at the end of the program, to remind the patients of the whole program content.

Many bipolar patients tend to organize their time rather erratically, although regularity would help them keep their disorder compensated. Regular schedules and better structuring of activities must thus be one of the key points in any individual intervention with a bipolar patient. In the group, all we can do is to get across the importance of these aspects, presenting them as information, as there is not enough time to work on techniques such as recording activities, which are usually useful for bipolar patients. It is important for patients to keep the proper balance between a schedule that maintains their euthymia and schedules that favor social adequacy and quality of life. In the case of very young patients, for example, keeping up a social network (another important aspect of the disorder) is far easier if the patient can go out some nights, but this behavior seems to run counter to stability of scheduling; the answer is to work out the proper balance between the two needs. It is important to attend to the individual needs of each patient, something that can only be done sketchily in the group setting.

Once again, it should be emphasized that our program does not claim to offer specific training in these skills, especially in the case of stress-management techniques; all we can do is make the patient aware of a number of techniques that may be useful at some point in time.

# Regularity of habits

## Goal

The goal of this session is to enter into greater depth on a point that has come up indirectly in almost all the sessions: the need for regular habits. Although this point is of extraordinary importance, we do not spend more time on it because it is a vital part of the work of the individual clinician.

## Procedure

- After the informal conversation, we can start the session by going through people's "fire extinguisher cards" and make the necessary corrections.
- We continue the session with the following story:

### The story of a bet

Alan and Guy happened to meet at the mall. At first they hardly noticed each other because the Christmas shopping rush was on and the downtown area was crowded at seven in the evening. They were thrilled to run into each other, as they had been out of touch for several months. They sat down in a café. Alan ordered a soft drink and Guy ordered a regular coffee. They remembered when they first met, in a psychiatric ward to which Alan had been taken involuntarily in a manic, psychotic state while Guy was recovering from a severe depressive episode. They became good friends, possibly because they were the only bipolars on the ward. In a joking tone, some patients had started to call them "the one" and "the two" referring to their diagnostic subtype and an overheard conversation between a very young doctor and a veteran nurse. So Alan was "the one" and Guy was "the two." They also called them "Groucho and Harpo" because Alan was very talkative, in contrast to Guy who rarely talk a single word. They both laughed over these anecdotes. Alan recounted that when he was discharged from the psychiatric ward he had been very tired for several weeks, but gradually felt better and was tolerating his lithium treatment well; this allowed him to return to his job as a civil servant and work on his relationship with his wife which was improving as she learned to understand his disorder. He now led a quiet life, played soccer on Wednesday afternoons, and spent the weekends looking after his wife, who was 7-month pregnant. Because of the pregnancy, they had moved to a very large apartment downtown, a little noisy but very spacious. Everything was going smoothly. He was worried only about a slight overweight problem, which is why he played soccer, took saunas, swallowed some slimming pills, and was on a diet that, although he found it a little tough, was helping him recover his self-esteem. Guy ordered another coffee and told his story. He was not doing too badly, either; he had recovered from his depression and had been taking his medication regularly ever since. He went out on Saturday nights, but, in order not to mix his medication with the little alcohol he drank, skipped the pill until the next morning. He worked as a waiter in a pizzeria and had chosen the night shift which paid better – he wanted to take a trip to Kenya – kept up his studies in the morning, and spent the afternoon on his great love, the piano. They both rejoiced that their lives had gone back to normal after the hospital stay, although the doctor had made it very clear that they were exposed to the risk of a relapse. After joking about it, they made a bet: they would meet up on the first Friday of the month at the same coffee shop and catch up. The first one to suffer a relapse would treat the other one to the movies. With a brief hug they said goodbye, both hoping to lose the bet so that it would be a long time before they went to the movies together.

*Question: Although we cannot read the future, which of them has the greater number of risk factors?*

- We ask the patients which of the two men in the story has the best chance of still being euthymic after a year, and why.
- The patients have to debate and list the risk factors for each of the patients in the story. The therapist uses the opportunity to comment, especially on habits.
- The story is seasoned with references to risk factors of greater or lesser importance, although it does not say which factors outweigh the others. The story was written to generate controversy and debate among the patients.
- The discussion of the issue serves as an introduction to the session material.

- If the story of the two men is not getting the point across to patients, we can send them to Example 5 in Session 6 (see p. 96) and repeat the life chart to emphasize the importance of regular habits.
- Before giving out the advice on sleep health, it is a good idea to let the patients themselves talk about their personal techniques, which are often very useful and original.
- We distribute the materials and end the session.

## Useful tips

- Our advice on the therapeutic use of sleep does not at any time touch on the use of sleep deprivation as a possible therapy for bipolar depression. The few studies that exist do not demonstrate that this technique has any long-term efficacy in treatment of bipolar disorders, although it is clear that the simple behavioral tip of reducing sleeping hours during depression is effective.
- Continuing with the sleep advice, we have to remember that this depends a great deal on learned habits and sometimes it is better to respect these habits, unless they are very disruptive, than try to change them. This is the case of patients who are heavy smokers, who cannot do without the last cigaret 5 min before falling asleep, or people who drop off in front of the TV. However, we cannot be permissive with other unhealthy habits such as coffee drinking or cannabis intake.
- In some cases it is a good idea to ask the patients to keep a sleep diary for a few months, so that they can become aware of any sleeping problems.
- With regard to diet, many of our patients are worried about their weight gain as many of them binge when they are anxious, or are sedentary; also some psychoactive drugs affect weight. It is advisable for a bipolar patient never to go on a very strict diet which involves going hungry, and in any case it is advisable for the diet to be monitored by a dietician and a psychologist.
- Many of our patients do not make rational use of sports and simply exercise when they feel like it – which is usually when they are starting to be hypomanic, and exercise makes things worse. We have to spend a few minutes explaining to our patients that sport is very desirable, especially if they are euthymic or depressed (we add that we know how much of an effort it is to play sports when one is depressed, but that it is usually very

good for combating the depression) but that sports are not advisable during a hypomanic or manic phase, or if the patient suspects that one of these phases is starting up. This information is often new to our patients, who have the idea that sports are always healthy. We emphasize that physical exercise during hypomania only makes the situation worse, due to overstimulation. We have to get across the idea that one should never try to head off hypomania or mania by exhaustion.

## Patient material

In all the prior sessions, we have placed a great deal of emphasis on regular habits. Regular sleep is probably one of the foundations of mood stability, because sleep has a twin function for a bipolar patient:

- Observing how we sleep can give us information on the status of our bipolar disorder: if we are only sleeping a little we are probably verging on hypomania, while if we tend to oversleep we are probably verging on a depression.
- We can use this information to help us: if we notice we are starting to feel depressed, it may be useful to reduce the number of sleep hours to improve our mood. On the other hand, a good way to head off a hypomanic decompensation is to make sure we are sleeping a good number of hours for a few days.

An adult should sleep between 7 and 9 h a day to repair physical and mental wear and tear and feel refreshed the next day. These hours should be sequential and at night, so that sleeping 5 h and taking a 2 h siesta to add up to 7 h is not a good idea. This is true regardless of whether or not one has bipolar disorder: apart from producing fatigue and physical malaise, sleeping poorly or cutting into sleep time causes irritability and memory problems, among many other problems.

Ideally, sleep hours should be regular throughout the week and one should avoid sleeping late at weekends – this may have direct effects on the quality of sleep during the week. However, if we go out and have a late night, it is a good idea to sleep the full 8 h even if this means not getting up until noon. It is agreed that such a serious disruption of the schedule should be the exception and not the rule. How often one can go out at night varies for each patient depending on their symptoms, the type of relapse that is most frequent, and the tolerance to this kind of disruption – all these depend on the individual.

"Pulling an all-nighter" because we are working, studying, or dancing is out of the question for a person suffering from bipolar disorder. A number of studies have shown that getting a little sleep for two nights in succession is enough to trigger a manic episode. Some patients have suffered a relapse after spending the whole night studying, so academic life should be planned ahead so as to avoid last-minute sprints (which do not give the best results anyway).

Regarding the siesta or afternoon nap: the maximum recommended time is about 30 min, and only if this does not affect nighttime sleep. We should never nap in the daytime if we suspect we are verging on a depression, and in no case should we undress and go to bed in the daytime. At most, we should take a little snooze, thus avoiding to watch the after-lunch soap opera (which is usually terrible anyway, with an incestuous, tangled plot).

Some tips to encourage what professionals call "sleep health" may help the patient get quality sleep:

- Go to bed only to sleep (or for sex, if you and your partner find this is appropriate). It is not advisable to use the bed for studying, watching TV, or eating, although it is acceptable to read before dropping off.
- Keep the room well ventilated during the day.
- Be sure not to eat heavy meals.
- Avoid chocolate and coffee, which are stimulants.
- If you smoke, the last cigaret should be smoked at the latest of half an hour before bedtime, as tobacco is a stimulant.
- During the last half hour before bedtime, it is not advisable to have the computer or TV on, as the light from the screen is a stimulant.
- If you work late, spend an hour unwinding with a relaxing activity such as reading or listening to music before going to bed.
- Try not to have an argument before going to bed (ideally, try not to have arguments!).
- Do not use an illuminated clock because you tend to watch the time passing and worry about how long it is taking to drop off – which only increases anxiety.

It is desirable for people suffering bipolar disorders to have a job with a strict habit schedule, hence jobs with constant shift changes, or no schedule, are not advisable. If a bipolar patient has a job requiring a lot of night work (doctor, nurse, fireman, policeman, waiter, etc.), he should try to stay off the night shift, submitting a medical report if necessary.

As far as food is concerned, we have some tips:

- Patients who are on lithium should not start a low-salt or salt-free diet suddenly (see material in Sessions 7 and 10, p. 111 and 126).
- Patients taking monoamine oxidase (MAO) inhibitor antidepressants should keep to the proper diet for these drugs (see Session 9, p. 122).
- In no case should one be on a strict diet: going hungry is very stressful and can even trigger a phase.
- Some bipolar patients often act out by "binging" – compulsively bolting down a large amount of food with the conscious or unconscious intention of soothing anxiety (generally carbohydrates, sweets, candy, or snacks such as French fries, almonds, etc.) If you notice binging behavior, you should tell the psychiatrist about it and seek treatment (there are good psycho-logical treatments for this type of problem).

Doing physical exercise is highly advisable for a person suffering from bipolar disorder, but we must bear in mind that sports are highly stimulat-ing, so it is best to practice sports during euthymia and, still better, during a depressive phase even though one does not feel like it. On the other hand, it is inadvisable to do sports during a hypomanic or manic phase, or if we sus-pect we are going into decompensation of this type. Remember: in these cases, physical activity is a natural antidepressant, but may make hypomanic or manic symptoms worse.

# Stress-control techniques

## Goal

Although stress is not a central or core topic in bipolar disorders, it clearly plays an important role in triggering episodes, especially the early episodes – it seems gradually to lose its power with subsequent relapses. Hence it should definitely be included in a psychoeducation program for bipolar disorders. There are two (modest) goals for this nineteenth session: emphasize the importance of stress as a trigger for relapses, and talk about the breadth of the stress concept, which patients normally associate only with job pressures. Also, we try to give our patients information on the existence of various psychological tools that can help them to manage stress and anxiety better. We do not try to train the patient in these techniques during the session, although at one time we tried including an initial training in muscle relaxation. We later saw that this was not very useful for many of our patients and might even confuse some of them. The only thing we are trying to do is to inform the patient about a tool that could be advisable in certain cases.

## Procedure

- As usual, we begin the session with an informal chat – which happens quite spontaneously by this stage in the program (in fact some effort has to be made by the therapists in the last three or four sessions to interrupt the group conversation rather than start it).
- We go over the distinction between causes and triggers (see Session 3, p. 73). A good way of doing this is to ask the group an open question about this difference and wait for answers before starting our explanation.
- We then explain the concept of stress using the session material.
- We look for examples of a clear psychosocial trigger from the patients themselves. At the same time, using some of the examples, we once again warn

against the risk of making wrong causal attributions or confusing cause and example, as in the case of a patient who said that he became depressed because he made a serious mistake at his job, although it may actually be the case that this serious mistake was related to the attentional and general functioning problems inherent in the beginning of a depressive phase.

- We can draw a life chart so that the patients can clearly see the relationship between stressor stimuli, both positive and negative, and relapses.
- If we have enough time, we can explain the controlled breathing technique (in a brief and practical way) just, hence the patients do not see these techniques as something mysterious or magical. We can ask a volunteer to try out the technique, or do it as a group exercise – something that many group members find entertaining, although it will probably not be useful in active prevention of anxiety.

## Useful tips

- An explanation of the stress concept can be rather tedious if it is not illustrated with constant examples.
- To avoid having patients make excessively psychologistic or simplistic attributions, it is important for them to understand that there are biochemical factors, cortisol for example, that are essential as mediators between stress and the possible start of decompensation.
- One thing that surprises patients and at the same time gives them a good measure for what was discussed in the previous point is the possibility that an apparently positive stress can treat a depressive phase and, conversely, a clearly negative stressor can trigger a (hypo)manic episode. It is interesting to search out moments in which group members were in this situation.
- We must make sure that the patients learn that stress is a broad concept and actually in our case refers to positive or negative overstimulation by the environment, as the majority of patients have a very limited concept of the word "stress."

## Patient material

The term "stress" is one of those that probably has a wider meaning if we look at what it means to the professional by comparison to what it means for the population at large. Most people understand the term "stress" as being trapped in several troublesome activities. In health science, on the other hand, we define stress as the sum of non-specific changes in the body with respect to a stimulus. Stress is an automatic response of the body to any change in the outer or inner environment, a response that prepares the body to deal with the possible demands generated by the new situation. This implies a significant increase in the level of physiological, motor, and cognitive activation.

Hence, stress depends both on the stimulus and on its perception by the individual and their resources for dealing with it. Some stimuli are experienced by some people as highly stressful, while for others they are quite ordinary. This is the case, for example, for speaking in public or driving at high speeds, which is absolutely not stressful for a professional driver but is for anyone else. In principle, the overactivation involved in the stress response is positive, as it enables the individual to meet the demands of the environment, but once some time has elapsed it has a disorganizing effect on behavior because the body can be overactivated for too long. Chronic, sustained overactivation can result in physical and mental problems: hypertension, asthma, insomnia, gastric problems, anxiety, depression, fatigue, tremors, etc.

The physiologic response to stress generally involves physiologic and activation and consists of three phases:

1 *Alarm phase*: Intense, immediate physiologic activation providing resources for possible action. If the stressful situation is overcome, the general activation syndrome ends; if not, phase B follows.
2 *Resistance phase*: Activation is maintained, less than in phase A but more than in normal. If the stressful situation is overcome, the general activation syndrome ends; if not, phase C follows.
3 *Exhaustion phase*: The body uses up its resources and suddenly loses its activation capacity.

A sustained stress situation has extremely damaging consequences for everyone, but especially someone suffering from bipolar disorder. Stress can lead to decompensation through two pathways:

1 *Directly*: The physiologic alteration itself causes changes in hormones and neurotransmitters, which can cause decompensation.

2  *Indirectly*: The stress acts negatively on basic areas such as sleep, and this in turn causes decompensation.

It is very important to point out that the sign of the stressor (positive or negative) is not necessarily the sign of the decompensation: a highly positive stimulus may trigger a depressive phase and a highly negative stimulus may give rise to a manic phase (as in the case of patients who start a manic phase after the death of a loved one).

It is advisable to try to stop or relieve stress before it causes a relapse. There are various techniques for doing this, which for convenience we summarize in Chart 3.

---

**Chart 3    How to deal with stress**

- *Rationalizing problems*: Most of the time we tend to overvalue things that concern us. Circumstances that are relatively banal in comparison what is truly important in life may overwhelm us if we do not put them in perspective. The world is not going to come to an end if we fail an exam or miss a job promotion. A psychologist can give us the proper tools for appropriately channeling our concerns.
- *Relaxation*: For many patients, it is useful to learn a relaxation technique and how to apply it when necessary, sometimes on a regular basis. The most widely used relaxation techniques are Jacobson's muscle relaxation and Schulz relaxation – less body-centered and focusing more on thought control. Either of these may be valuable for a person who is prone to anxiety or is exposed to stressors.
- *Breath control*: In many stressful situations, it is not possible to relax as this is a technique that requires some time, training and a proper space. Learning controlled or diaphragmatic breathing can be very useful for these situations, apart from which it is a technique much used by people who work with the voice and need high-quality breathing.

# Problem-solving strategies

## Goal

As with the last session, we do not view problem-solving as an essential topic in the psychoeducation of a bipolar patient; nonetheless, decision-making is complex for people who suffer this disorder once they have learned not to make decisions when they are sick, or on the spur of the moment. Patients like this type of session because they understand they are acquiring tools that go beyond learning about the disorder. Little by little, this particular session has evolved, and we now use it in our groups to deal with the real, daily problems of an individual suffering bipolar disorder: deciding who to tell about the disorder, what employment or academic limits should be set or imposed – if we have to impose them ourselves – how to plan the daily routine so that it is less stressful, or how to plan our vacations. The last issue has shown up in all the groups we have run so far, so that we decided to prepare material to deal with it, hence patients have something concrete to hold onto. Once again, our program does not claim to be a structured training in problem-solving techniques, which would take several sessions. Our intention is just to sketch out ways of structuring the decision-making process.

## Procedure

- Once the group has stopped chatting and we have some minimal attention, we explain why we are devoting a session to problem-solving techniques.
- We briefly present the theoretical problem-solving model.
- We ask the group to come up with an invented problem so that we can apply the technique as a group.
- We define the problem operationally. It is interesting that, for this step and the next ones, we use the blackboard: we have to note each step so that the patient understands how easy it is to work with written material in decision-making.

- We "brainstorm" the problem as a group, making sure all the patients participate.
- To evaluate the probability of solving the problem, the emotional response, the time and effort it requires, and the long-term effects, we can vote among the group, while making it clear that psychoeducation actually has to be done on an individual basis.
- We can spend about 40 min on psychoeducation and half an hour on preparing to make trips.
- We ask the patients something like "Imagine you are going on a trip … What could turn out badly?" Everyone in turn has a chance to respond, and we do not need the blackboard for this step.
- Once we have joked about things like the plane crashing (someone always brings up this possibility – i.e., an earthquake at our destination) we can go on to talk about preventive behavior when planning a trip.
- Then we open the group up to discussion and questions, after which we conclude the session.

## Useful tips

- When brainstorming, it is appropriate for the therapist not to give the idea that they are invested with any authority or they risk having their solution being overevaluated as the best one, which prevents the technique from being properly used. If the therapist comes up with a solution, it must be obviously absurd and amusing, to remind the patients of the need to include *all types of solutions* when brainstorming.
- It is important to make it clear to the patients that we are only teaching them a framework for a possible decision-making method, which in no event must replace their common sense. The risk of cognitive–behavioral techniques, especially if applied by an inexperienced psychologist, is that the patient feels undervalued by the therapist, that is if patients feel that their psychologist thinks they are fools. We always have to point out that we are only demonstrating one more resource for decision-making.
- About travel: some patients may interpret our advice as a way of creating obstacles to bipolars traveling, or a veiled way of advising them against travel. We have to explain this point.

## Patient material

### Problem-solving

- It is impossible not to have problems. In fact, life usually consists of solving a series of small or large problems, alternating with moments of satisfaction (which are often related to the solving of a problem). Anyone, whether diagnosed or not, has many problems or decision points every day, from the simplest questions (What shall I wear today? What shall I have for breakfast? Which way shall I go to work?) up to very complex decisions (Should I fire an employee? Should I move house? Get divorced? Stay on at school?). Complex decisions may be very stressful, undermine the quality of life of the decision-maker, and, in the case of a person with bipolar disorder, trigger a period of anxiety and insomnia which, as we already know, can lead to an episode. We must remember that in no event should important decisions be made when there is a suspicion (because we have detected warning signs) or conviction (because the psychiatrist has told us) that we are going into decompensation, of whatever type, and that decisions should always be taken in a euthymic mood, that is without symptoms *per se*. Many bipolar patients have difficulty solving problems or making decisions, so learning a few tricks can be beneficial. The process to use is as follows:
- The first thing to bear in mind is that the majority of problems or important decisions should be taken slowly. Haste and impulsivity are poor guides. The first step in our problem-solving plan is to *inhibit the tendency to respond impulsively to a* problem. Whenever possible, we need to give ourselves time to make an important decision. This will allow us to:
  - Gather objective, relevant information about the problem.
  - Understand the conflict, that is understand the gap between where I am now and where I want to be, what are the conditions for change, and what obstacles I will meet on the way.
  - Define realistic, concrete objectives.
  - Evaluate the short- and long-term benefits and costs.
- The second step in decision-making or problem-solving is to *generate as many answers as* possible even through we are obviously not going to use all of them and some of them may be unsuitable or even nutty. To generate these answers we use a technique called "brainstorming" which is spontaneously coming up with as many alternatives as possible, writing

them down, then evaluating them. There are three basic rules with this technique:

1 *Quantity principle*: come up with as many solutions as possible.
2 *Postponing judgment principle*: everything is equally valid. We are not trying here to evaluate the quality or possible effectiveness of the alternatives we generate, because this is step three.
3 *Variety principle*: the alternatives should be as multicolored as possible, avoiding conventionalisms and repeating alternatives that go along the same lines as others.

- The third step is to establish a procedure for *choosing the most appropriate* response out of all the responses generated. From the long list of solutions, we must now choose the solution that brings us the most benefit at the lowest cost. The solution must be *effective* for reaching our objectives, and must also be *possible*. We evaluate each alternative generated against the following:
  - The probability that this alternative will resolve the conflict (we can assign a score if this is difficult).
  - The emotional response it generates: does it reduce our anxiety or does it give us a sense of ease?
  - The time and effort it requires.
  - Its long-term effects.

If we have scored each of these factors, we need only to add up the scores to see which solution is the most workable.

Of course, this is a very mechanical and artificial way of making decisions, and just gives us a controlled way of making decisions to reduce anxiety. Applying this pencil-and-paper method a couple of times will help us to integrate this as a part of our daily functioning, without needing to go through the procedure explicitly each time, but keeping it for "major occasions."

## Planning a trip

A trip, whether for a vacation or for rest, can be stressful for anyone who is not properly organized. For people who suffer from bipolar disorders, the following points must be borne in mind:

- We should always plan the trip when in a state of euthymia: never during a depression, "to run away," or during hypomania or mania. At most, we could make a trip when slightly depressed.

- We always take with us *triple the medication* we need. If a patient is taking three lithium tablets and one lorazepam tablet, and going on a 10-day trip, he should bring along three different pill boxes, each containing 30 lithium tablets and 10 lorazepam.
- During the trip, put the three pill boxes in three different places, for example one in the carry-on bag (the bag we keep with us on the airplane), another in the checked luggage, and another in one's jacket, so that if the other two are lost we still have enough medication. We also bring along *rescue medication*, that is what we have to take if we suspect a hypomanic phase is starting.
- The psychiatrist should write a *report in English* – regardless of their native language – explaining the diagnosis and type of treatment the patient is taking. It is important not to use trade names when describing the treatment, but active principles (venlafaxine, oxycarbazepine, lorazepam) as trade names often vary from one country to another.
- Always bring along the telephone number and address of our citizenship embassy at our destination.
- About *jet lag*: the advice given is always to adjust as soon as possible to the time zone of the destination; we start when we get on the plane by setting our watch to the current time at our destination. Once there, we try to be consistent with this time change, bearing in mind that it is generally better to sleep too much than too little on the flight. The medication prescribed by the psychiatrist may make it easier to sleep. Sometimes, a face mask and ear plugs may be used to make it easier to drop off on the plane.
- We must remember that vacations are for *resting*. We cannot see Rome in one day, Paris in two, New York in three, or Peru in four, because this would obviously be too stressful.

# Session 21

# Closure

## Goal

Session number 21 will be used to close the group properly. The experience of sharing a program for 20 weeks usually creates strong bonds between patients, and between the patients and the group as a whole, so that for them the act of closure has a strong emotional value.

## Procedure

- We can use the first half hour to resolve any doubts about the material from previous sessions.
- The next step is to ask the group how they believe their participation in the program has changed their behavior or way of thinking with respect to various areas:
  - Awareness of the disorder.
  - Need for treatment.
  - Detection of symptoms.
  - Suicidal thinking.
  - How to explain the disorder to friends and acquaintances.
  - How to structure time.
  - Taking toxic substances.
- This point is especially important because, on the one hand, it allows us to make some kind of evaluation of the subjective benefit to our patients, and on the other hand it allows us to establish some content.
- The next step is to ask the patients to evaluate the program. This can be done as follows:

"Between the time we started this type of program 10-years ago and the present, we think we have done a great deal to improve its quality. This is largely because two of us professionals now have more experience, but even more because of the changes we have incorporated following your comments and suggestions. Without constructive criticism, we cannot move forward. Please be as honest and direct as possible: What can we do to improve our program? Do you think anything is missing or should be pruned? Was any of the program more than you needed?"

- This usually starts a round of comment, most of it very sincere. The vast majority of people who have completed the program enjoy it; most say they became a little bored with "so many sessions on medication," but despite this they wished the program would go on for longer.
- In the same round, each patient can explain how he feels.
- We give a material with a Bibliography (see p. 200) so that they can stay informed about bipolar disorders.
- We thank the group, and say our goodbyes.

## Useful tips

- Perhaps the most important point of the last session is to avoid leaving patients feeling "high and dry" when the program ends, as many of them have lived in a "safety zone" from the communicative and affective standpoint, apart from the usefulness of its content. For this reason, it is important to leave the door open to consultation once the program is over, meaning that we should give the patients our office number at the center, our professional phone number, our office hours, and, above all, the feeling of availability.
- Many patients ask to exchange phone numbers, addresses, and e-mail addresses with other patients. Although this is a majority choice of the group and a positive reflection of the level of bonding, the therapist should not lead this initiative in any way or make it official, as this could be very upsetting for a patient who is not disposed to staying in touch with others in the program.
- Before the group is concluded, we publicly thank its members for staying with the program to the end and for respecting group rules. We express our gratitude for facilitating our work, provided this gratitude is authentic

and clear. At the door we shake hands with all the patients as we say good-bye, so that our leave-taking is not only *public* but *personal.*

## And after the group … what?

Although in the many lectures and courses we have given around the world, many professionals complain that our program lasts too long and that it is very difficult for bipolar patients to comply with such a long program, or that this type of program could be incorporated into normal clinical practice, our patients complain that the program is too short and that there is no follow-up. In fact, they complain that they are suddenly "support orphans." Of course, they have all been informed ahead of time that the psychoeducation program is time limited, and during the group we do everything possible to generate autonomous behavior in our patients and prevent dependency, but it is almost inevitable that if they enjoyed the program they will want to prolong the enjoyment. We have several times discussed the possibility of booster sessions after a certain amount of time, not so much for the reasons given above but so that we can check on the prophylactic efficacy of our intervention. This is something we have not been able to do so far, but it could make sense. An intervention that is possible, valuable, and effective is to continue the work started in the group with individual cognitive–behavioral therapy, something which is necessary for many patients. Our work would consist of helping the patient find stress management courses, facilitate the handling of symptoms, and deal with the psychosocial epiphenomena of the disorder itself. However, these options are by no means essential as many of our patients achieve sufficient behavioral change just by participating in the psychoeducation program.

## Patient material

### Staying informed

You are now actually experts in bipolar disorders and, what is more important, *your bipolar disorder.* Congratulations. If you are curious enough to read more, here are some informational books we can recommend. We do recommend that you stay away from technical books for psychiatrists, psychologists, and other professionals, which often use language that is difficult for non-health-professionals to understand. You should also avoid easy "recipe" books for "improving as a person," based on unscientific beliefs. We recommend:

Torrey, E.F., and Knable, M.B.: *Surviving Manic-Depression.* New York: Basic Books, 2002.
Miklowitz, D.J.: The Bipolar Disorder Survival Guide. New York: Guilford Press, 2002.
Scott, J. Overcoming Your Mood-Swings. London: Robinson, 2001.

# Final note:
# Is psychoeducation efficacious?

Although much clinicians have used psychoeducation for decades, it has not been until a few years ago that the first studies on its efficacy came out. The studies by Peet and Harvey may be considered the first to evaluate the efficacy of psychoeducation (Harvey and Peet, 1991; Peet and Harvey, 1991). They formed two groups of 30 bipolar patients; the first group was shown a 12-min video giving information on lithium and the patients were given a transcript of the text, while the second group acted as a control group and received standard treatment. The attitudes of the patients toward lithium and their knowledge about the treatment improved significantly in the first group.

Van Gent and Zwart (1991) compared 14 bipolar patients who received five group psychoeducation sessions with another 12 patients who acted as the control group. Although the first group showed better knowledge of the disorder and the medication, and better social skills, no effect on treatment adherence was observed. In later studies, the same research group found a significant drop in non-adherence and number of hospital admissions in the group receiving psychoeducation (Van Gent, 2000). It is interesting to note the great tradition of psychoeducation in the Netherlands, at least from the standpoint of clinical support, a tradition that led to its inclusion in the clinical practice routines of many hospitals and favored development of the Netherlands' own psychoeducation group model – very short in duration, and emphasizing collaboration in the psychiatrist–patient relationship.

In many patients with some type of psychosis, there is evidence of the efficacy of psychological intervention in improving adherence (Kemp et al., 1996). The approach tested in this article, which appeared in the prestigious *British Medical Journal*, was based on the motivational interview and cognitive intervention. Data on studies conducted exclusively with bipolar patients are somewhat scarce and less conclusive: the study by Cochran (1984) which measured the efficacy of adherence-centered cognitive intervention, offers results that are convincing but somewhat limited by the small sample size ($N = 28$). Other, later, studies suffer from the same defect (Scott and Tacchi, 2002). One good study from the methodological standpoint is that by Eduard Van Gent (1991): this is a brief psychoeducative intervention in pairs of bipolar patients which did not show efficacy in improving patient adherence. This result contrasts with a similar study (Clarkin et al., 1998) who, using similar methodology, obtained good adherence results. The only difference between the two interventions was how long they lasted: five sessions in the case of the Dutch group, and 11 months of treatment in the case of Clarkin. It is clear that sometimes shorter does not mean better.

Another basic strategy for achieving better prevention of relapses is to teach the patient to detect them early so that prompt intervention can occur. Here, there are very solid data from studies with adequate samples, highly structured treatments, and designs characterized by a very restrictive methodology. Perhaps the best study on individual psychological intervention in bipolar disorder is that by Perry et al. (1999) in which the type of intervention used included a variable number of sessions (between 7 and 12) during which the therapist, with a clearly psychoeducative approach, helped the patients identify their most usual relapse signals. The results indicated that the patients in the treatment group ($N = 34$) took longer to suffer a manic relapse and, at the end of the follow-up, had fewer manic relapses than the control group ($N = 35$). It seems that there was no effect at all in preventing depressive episodes.

The studies made by our group showed a solid effect of psychoeducation in preventing all types of episodes (Colom et al., 2003a) and hospitalization days. Our study was the first to show the prophylactic efficacy of group psychoeducation in a randomized trial, with evaluators blinded to the intervention, with an adequate sample ($N = 120$), and long-term follow-up (24 months). At 2 years, the type I or II bipolar patients who received psychoeducation and drug treatment suffered a significantly lower number of relapses than the patients in the control group, who received unstructured group intervention as a placebo in addition to drug treatment (Figure 9).

Now that the efficacy of psychoeducation had been demonstrated, the next logical step was to test how it worked and observe whether the effect was mediated only by improved adherence. To explore this, we designed a new study

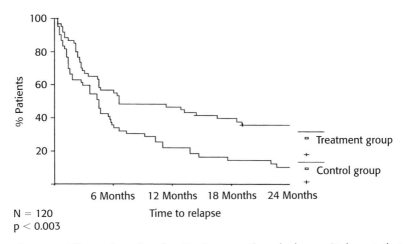

N = 120
p < 0.003

Figure 9    Efficacy of psychoeducation in prevention of relapses (Colom et al., *Arch Gen Psychiatry*, 2003a).

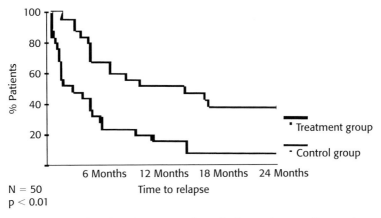

N = 50
p < 0.01

Figure 10    Psychoeducation: prevention of relapses in compliant patients with type I bipolar disorder (Colom et al., *J. Clin. Psychiatry*, 2003b).

with a somewhat smaller ($N = 50$) but more homogenous sample (only patients with type I bipolar disorders). The rest of the design was exactly the same as in the first study, except that we included only patients with good drug adherence to ensure that, if efficacy was observed, it would not be related to adherence improvement. At 2 years follow-up, psychoeducation also showed its efficacy in reducing the total number of relapses and preventing depressive relapses (Colom et al., 2003b), showing that the other units of the program also played an active role (Figure 10).

We are thus able to state that the prophylactic efficacy of psychoeducation in bipolar disorders has been demonstrated, which amply justifies its inclusion in normal clinical practice. This manual gives details of the intervention referred to in our group's article published in the prestigious journal *Archives of General Psychiatry*. Anyone who applies the techniques we describe in this text can expect a greater improvement in the course of the disorder in patients included in the group than could be expected with medication alone. We trust that this manual will allow many more patients to benefit from psychoeducation; thus, not only will the disorder go better, but they will be more free.

# Bibliography

Abraham, K.: Notes on the psychoanalytical investigation and treatment of manic-depressive insanity and allied conditions (1911). In: *Selected Papers of Karl Abraham, MD.* Translated by Bryan, D., and Strachey, A. London: Hogarth Press, 1927, pp. 137–156.

Adams, J., and Scott, J.: Predicting medication adherence in severe mental disorders. *Acta Psychiat Scand* 2000; 101: 119–24.

Akiskal, H.S.: El espectro clínico predominante de los trastornos bipolares [The predominant clinical spectrum of bipolar disorders]. In: Vieta, E., and Gasto, C. (eds.). *Trastornos Bipolares.* Barcelona: Springer-Verlag, 1997, pp. 194–212.

Akiskal, H.S., Bourgeois, M.L., Angst, J., Post, R., Moller, H., and Hirschfeld, R.: Reevaluating the prevalence of and diagnostic composition within the broad clinical spectrum of bipolar disorders. *J Affect Disord* 2000; 59 (Suppl 1): 5–30.

Angst, J.: Epidemiologie du spectre bipolaire [Epidemiology of the bipolar spectrum]. *Encephale* 1995; 21 (Suppl 6): 37–42.

Angst, J.: The emerging epidemiology of hypomania and bipolar II disorder. *J Affect Disord* 1998; 50: 143–151.

Angst, J., and Perris, C.: [On the nosology of endogenous depression. Comparision of the results of two studies]. *Arch Psychiat Nervenkr.* 1968; 210: 373–86.

Ayuso-Gutiérrez, J.L., and Ramos-Brieva, J.A.: The course of manic-depressive illness. A comparative study of bipolar I and bipolar II patients. *J Affect Disord* 1982, 4: 9–14.

Basco, M.R., and Rush, A.J.: *Cognitive–Behavioral Therapy for Bipolar Disorder.* New York: The Guilford Press, 1996.

Bauer, M.S.: An easy-access program for bipolar disorder. *Syllabus and Proceedings Summary of the 150th Annual Meeting of the American Psychiatric Association.* New York, 1997; 59.

Bauer, M.S., and McBride, L.: *Structured Group psychotherapy for Bipolar Disorder. The Life Goals Program.* New York: Springer Publishing Company, 1996.

Beck, A.T.: *Cognitive Theory and the Emotional Disorders.* New York: International Universities Press, 1976, pp. 47–132.

Beck, A.T., Rush, A.J., Shaw, B., and Emery, G.: *Cognitive Therapy of Depression.* New York: John Wiley & Sons, 1979.

Benazzi, F.: Is four days the minimum duration of hypomania in bipolar II disorder? *Eur Arch Psychiat Clin Neurosci* 2001; 251: 32–34.

Blackburn, I.M., and Moore, R.G.: Controlled acute and follow-up trial of cognitive therapy and pharmacotherapy in outpatients with recurrent depression. *Br J Psychiat* 1997; 171: 328–334.

**206**     **Bibliography**

Buckley, P., Cannon, M., and Larkin, C.: Abuse of neuroleptic drugs. *Br J Addict* 1991; 86: 789–790.

Chakrabarti, S., Kulhara, P., and Verma, S.K.: Extent and determinants of burden among families of patients with affective disorders. *Acta Psychiat Scand* 1992; 86: 247–252.

Clarkin, J.F., Carpenter, D., Hull, J., Wilner, P., and Glick, I.: Effects of psychoeducational intervention for married patients with bipolar disorder and their spouses. *Psychiat Serv* 1998; 49: 531–533.

Cochran, S.D.: Preventing medical nonadherence in outpatient treatment of bipolar disorders. *J Consult Clin Psychol* 1984; 52: 873–878.

Colom, F., Vieta, E., Martinez-Arán, A., Reinares, M., Benabarre, A., and Gastó, C.: Clinical factors associated to treatment nonadherence in euthymic bipolar patients. *J Clin Psychiat* 2000; 61: 549–554.

Colom, F., Vieta, E., Benabarre, A., Martinez-Arán, A., Reinares, M., Corbella, B., and Gasto, C.: Topiramate abuse in a bipolar patient with an eating disorder. *J Clin Psychiat* 2001; 62: 475–476.

Colom, F., Martinez-Arán, A., Reinares, M., Torrent, C., and Vieta, E.: Las cogniciones hipomaniacas [Hypomanic cognitions]. In: Vieta, E. (ed.). *Hipomania*, Madrid: Aula Médica, 2002.

Colom, F., Vieta, E., Martinez-Arán, A., Reinares, M., Goikolea, J.M., Benabarre, A., Torrent, C., Comes, M., Corbella, B., Parramon, G., and Corominas, J.: A randomized trial on the efficacy of group psychoeducation in the prophylaxis of recurrences in bipolar patients whose disease is in remission. *Arch Gen Psychiat* 2003a; 60: 402–407.

Colom, F., Vieta, E., Reinares, M., Martinez-Arán, A., Torrent, C., Goikolea, J.M., and Gastó, C.: Psychoeducation efficacy in bipolar disorders beyond adherence enhancement. *J Clin Psychiat* 2003b; 64: 1101–1105.

Coryell, W., Endicott, J., Maser, J.D., Keller, M.B., Leon, A.C., and Akiskal, H.S.: Long-term stability of polarity distinctions in the affective disorders. *Am J Psychiat* 1995; 152: 385–390.

Davenport, Y.B., Ebert, M.H., Adland, M.L., and Goodwin, F.H.: Couples group therapy as an adjunct to lithium maintenance of the manic patient. *Am J Orthopsychiat* 1977; 47: 495–502.

Delisie, J.D.: A case of amitriptyline abuse. *Am J Psychiat* 1990; 147: 1377–1378.

Dore, G., and Romans, S.E.: Impact of bipolar affective disorder on family and partners. *J Affect Disord* 2001; 67: 147–158.

Dunner, D.L.: Unipolar and bipolar depression: recent findings from clinical and biologic studies. In: *The Psychobiology of Affective Disorders. Pfizer Symposium on Depression.* Basel: Karger, 1980; pp. 11–24.

Ehlers, C.L., Frank, E., and Kupfer, D.J.: Social zeitgebers and biological rhythms: a unified approach to understanding the etiology of depression. *Arch Gen Psychiat* 1988; 45: 948–952.

Fava, G.A., Grandi, S., Zielezny, M., Rafanelli, C., and Canestrari, R.: Four-year outcome for cognitive–behavioral treatment of residual symptoms in major depression. *Am J Psychiat* 1996; 153: 945–947.

Fava, G.A., Savron, G., Grandi, S., and Rafanelli, C.: Cognitive–behavioral management of drug-resistant major depressive disorder. *J Clin Psychiat* 1997; 58: 278–282.

Fava, G.A., Rafanelli, C., Grandi, S., Conti, S., and Belluardo, P.: Prevention of recurrent depression with cognitive–behavioral therapy: preliminary findings. *Arch Gen Psychiat* 1998; 55: 816–820.

Fava, G.A., Bartolucci, G., Rafanelli, C., and Mangelli, L.: Cognitive–behavioral management of patients with bipolar disorder who relapsed while on lithium prophylaxis. *J Clin Psychiat* 2001; 62: 556–559.

Foelker, G.A., Molinari, V., Marmion, J.J., and Chacko, R.C.: Lithium groups and elderly bipolar outpatients. *Clin Gerontol* 1986; 5: 297–307.

Frank, E., Kupfer, D.J., Perel, J.M., Cornes, C., Jarret, D.B., Mallinger, A.G., Thase, M.E., McEachran, A.B., and Grochocinski, V.J.: Three-year outcome for maintenance therapies in recurrent depression. *Arch Gen Psychiat* 1990; 47: 1093–1099.

Frank, E., Kupfer, D.J., Wagner, E.F., McEachran, A.B., and Cornes, C.: Efficacy of interpersonal psychotherapy as a maintenance treatment of recurrent depression: contributing factors. *Arch Gen Psychiat* 1991; 48: 1053–1059.

Frank, E., Kupfer, D.J., Ehlers, C.L., Monk, T.H., Cornes, C., Carter, S., and Frankel D.: Interpersonal and social rhythm therapy for bipolar disorder: integrating interpersonal and behavioral approaches. *Behav Ther* 1994; 17: 153–156.

Frank, E., Swartz, H.A., and Kupfer, D.J.: Interpersonal and social rhythm therapy: managing the chaos of bipolar disorder. *Biol Psychiat* 2000; 48: 593–604.

Goetzel, R.Z., Hawkins, K., Ozminkowski, R.J., and Wang, S.: The health and productivity cost burden of the "top 10" physical and mental health conditions affecting six large US employers in 1999. *J Occup Environ Med* 2003; 45: 5–14.

Goodwin, F.K., and Jamison, R.: *Manic-Depressive Illness.* New York: Oxford University Press, 1990.

Graves, J.S.: Living with mania: a study of outpatient group psychotherapy for bipolar patients. *Am J Psychother* 1993; 47: 113–126.

Harvey, N.S., and Peet, M.: Lithium maintenance: effects of personality and attitude on health information acquisition and adherence. *Br J Psychiat* 1991; 158: 200–204.

Hirschfeld, R.M., Calabrese, J.R., Weissman, M.M., Reed, M., Davies, M.A., Frye, M.A., Keck Jr., P.E., Lewis, L., McElroy, S.L., McNulty, J.P., and Wagner, K.D.: Screening for bipolar disorder in the community. *J Clin Psychiat* 2003; 64: 53–59.

Jacobs, L.I.: Cognitive therapy of post-manic and post-depressive dysphoria in bipolar illness. *Am J Psychother* 1982; 36: 450–458.

Jamison, K.R., Gerner, R.H., and Goodwin, F.K.: Patient and physician attitudes toward lithium. *Arch Gen Psychiat* 1979; 36: 866–869.

Jarrett, R.B., Schaffer, M., McIntire, D., Witt-Browder, A., Kraft, D., and Risser, R.C.: Treatment of atypical depression with cognitive therapy or phenelzine: a double-blind, placebo-controlled trial. *Arch Gen Psychiat* 1999; 56: 431–437.

Jarrett, R.B., Kraft, D., Doyle, J., Foster, B.M., Eaves, G.G., and Silver, P.C.: Preventing recurrent depression using cognitive therapy with and without a continuation phase: a randomized clinical trial. *Arch Gen Psychiat* 2001; 58: 381–388.

Keller, M.B., McCullough, J.P., Klein, D.N., Arnow, B., Dunner, D.L., Gelenberg, A.J., Markowitz, J.C., Nemeroff, C.B., Russell, J.M., Thase, M.E., Trivedi, M.H., and Zajecka, J.: A comparison of nefazodone, the cognitive–behavioral analysis system of psychotherapy, and their combination for the treatment of chronic depression. *New Engl J Med* 2000; 342: 1462–1470.

Kemp, R., Hayward, P., and Applewhaite, G.: Adherence therapy in psychotic patients: randomized controlled trial. *Br Med J* 1996; 312: 345–349.

Kingdon, D., Farr, P., Murphy, S., and Tyrer, P.: Hypomania following cognitive therapy. *Br J Psychiat* 1986; 148: 103–104.

Kirmayer, L.J., and Groleau, D.: Affective disorders in cultural context. *Psychiat Clin North Am* 2001; 24: 465–478.

Klerman, G.L.: Principles of interpersonal psychotherapy for depression. In: Georgotas, A., and Cancro, R. (eds.). *Depression and Mania*. New York: Elsevier, 1988.

Klerman, G.L., Weissman, M.M., Rounsaville, B.J., and Chevron, E.S.: *Interpersonal Psychotherapy of Depression*. New York: Basic Books, 1984.

Kripke, D.F., and Robinson, D.: Ten years with a lithium group. *McLean Hosp J* 1985; 10: 1–11.

Kupfer, D.J., Franke, E., Perel, J.M., Cornes, C., Mallinger, A.G., Thase, M.E., McEachran, A.B., and Grochocinski, V.J.: Five-year outcome for maintenance therapies in recurrent depression. *Arch Gen Psychiat* 1992; 49: 769–773.

Lam, D., and Wong, B.: Prodromes, coping strategies, insight, and social functioning in bipolar affective disorders. *Psychol Med* 1997; 27: 1091–1100.

Lam, D.H., Jones, S.H., Hayward, P., and Bright, J.A.: *Cognitive Therapy for Bipolar Disorder*. Chichester: John Wiley & Sons Ltd., 1999.

Lam, D.H., Watkins, E.R., Hayward, P., Bright, J.A., Wright, K., Kerr, N., Parr-Davis, G., and Sham, P.: A randomized controlled study of cognitive therapy for relapse prevention for bipolar affective disorder. Outcome of the first year. *Arch Gen Psychiat* 2003; 60: 145–152.

Leahy, R.L., and Beck, A.T.: Cognitive therapy of depression and mania. In: Gorgotas, A., and Cancro, R. (eds.). *Depression and Mania*. New York: Elsevier, 1988.

López, A.D., and Murray, C.J.: The global burden of disease. *Nat Med* 1998; 4: 1241–1243.

Maj, M.: Lithium prophylaxis of bipolar disorder in ordinary clinical conditions: patterns of long-term outcome. In: Goldberg, J.F., and Harrow, M. (eds.). *Bipolar Disorders: Clinical Course and Outcome*. Washington, DC: American Psychiatric Press 1999, pp. 21–39.

McElroy, S., Keck Jr., P.E., and Strakowski, S.M.: Mania, psychosis, and antipsychotics. *J Clin Psychiat* 1996; 57 (Suppl 3): 14–26.

Menchón, J.M., Gastó, C., Vallejo, J., Catalán, R., Otero, A., and Vieta, E.: Rate and significance of hypomanic switches in unipolar melancholic depression. *Eur Psychiat* 1993; 8: 125–129.

Miklowitz, D.J., and Goldstein, M.J.: Behavioral family treatment for patients with bipolar affective disorder. *Behav Modif* 1990; 14: 457–489.

Miklowitz, D.J., Simoneau, T.L., George, E.L., Richards, J.A., Kalbag, A., Sachs-Ericsson, N., and Suddath, R.: Family-focused treatment of bipolar disorder: one-year effects of a psychoeducational program in conjunction with pharmacotherapy. *Biol Psychiat* 2000; 48: 582–592.

Miklowitz, D.J., George, E.L., Richards, J.A., Simoneau, T.L., and Suddath, R.L.: A randomized study of family-focused psychoeducation and pharmacotherapy in the outpatient management of bipolar disorder. *Arch Gen Psychiat* 2003; 60: 904–912.

Mitchell, P.B., and Malhi, G.S.: Treatment of bipolar depression: focus on pharmacologic therapies. *Expert Rev Neurother* 2005; 5: 69–78.

Morselli, P.L., and Elgie, R.: GAMIAN-Europe. GAMIAN-Europe/BEAM survey I-global analysis of a patient questionnaire circulated to 3450 members of twelve European advocacy groups operating in the field of mood disorders. *Bipolar Disord* 2003; 5: 265–278.

Murphy, F.C., Rubinsztein, J.S., Michael, A., Rogers, R.D., Robbins, T.W., Paykel, E.S., and Sahakian, B.J.: Decision-making cognition in mania and depression. *Psychol Med* 2001; 31: 679–693.

Palmer, A., and Williams, H.: CBT in a group format for bipolar affective disorder. *Beh Cogn Psychoth* 1995; 23: 153–168.

Patelis-Siotis, I., Young, L.T., Robb, J.C., Marriott, M., Bieling, P.J., Cox, L.C., and Joffe, R.T.: Group cognitive–behavioral therapy for bipolar disorder: a feasibility and effectiveness study. *J Affect Disord* 2001; 65: 145–153.

Paykel, E.S.: Psychotherapy, medication combinations, and adherence. *J Clin Psychiat* 1995; 56 (Suppl): 24–30.

Peet, M., and Harvey, N.S.: Lithium maintenance: I. A standard education program for patients. *Br J Psychiat* 1991; 158: 197–200.

Perlick, D., Clarkin, J.F., Sirey, J., Raue, P., Greenfield, S., Struening, E., and Rosenheck, R.: Burden experienced by care-givers of persons with bipolar-affective disorder. *Br J Psychiat* 1999; 175: 56–62.

Perlick, D.A., Rosenheck, R.R., Clarkin, J.F., Raue, P., and Sirey, P.H.: Impact of family burden and patient symptom status on clinical outcome in bipolar-affective disorder. *J Nerv Ment Dis* 2001; 189: 31–37.

Perlis, R.H., Nierenberg, A.A., Alpert, J.E., Pava, J., Matthews, J.D., Buchin, J., Sickinger, A.H., and Fava, M.: Effects of adding cognitive therapy to fluoxetine dose increase on risk of relapse and residual depressive symptoms in continuation treatment of major depressive disorder. *J Clin Psychopharm* 2002; 22: 474–480.

Perry, A., Tarrier, N., Morris, R., McCarthy, E., and Limb, K.: Randomized controlled trial of efficacy of teaching patients with bipolar disorder to identify early symptoms of relapse and obtain treatment. *Br Med J* 1999; 318: 149–153.

Pichot, O.: El nacimiento del trastorno bipolar [The birth of bipolar disorder]. *Eur Psychiat* (Sp. Ed.) 1995; 2: 143–158.

Pollack, L.E.: Treatment of inpatients with bipolar disorders: a role for self-management groups. *J Psychosoc Nurs* 1995; 33: 11–16.

Reinares, M., Colom, F., Martinez-Arán, A., Benabarre, A., and Vieta, E.: Therapeutic interventions focused on the family of bipolar patients. *Psychother Psychosom* 2002a; 71: 2–10.

Reinares, M., Vieta, E., Colom, F., Torrent, C., Comes, M., Benabarre, A., Goikolea, J.M., and Corbella, B.: Intervencion familiar de tipo psicoeducativo en el trastorno bipolar [Psychoeducational family intervention in bipolar disorder]. *Rev Psiquiatria Fac Med Barna* 2002b; 29(2): 97–105.

Reinares, M., Vieta, E., Colom, F., Martinez-Arán, A., Torrent, C., Comes, M., Goikolea, J.M., Benabarre, A., and Sánchez-Moreno, J.: Impact of a psychoeducational family intervention on caregivers of stabilized bipolar patients. *Psychother Psychsom* 2004; 73: 312–319.

Rosenfeld, H.: Notes on the psychopathology and psychoanalytic treatment of depressive and manic-depressive patients. In: Azima, H., and Glueck, B.C. (eds.). *Psychiatry Research Report* 17. Washington, DC: American Psychiatric Association 1963, pp. 73–83.

Scott, J., and Tacchi, M.J.: A pilot study of concordance therapy for individuals with bipolar disorders who are nonadherent with lithium prophylaxis. *Bipolar Disord* 2002; 4: 386–392.

Scott, J., Teasdale, J.D., Paykel, E.S., Johnson, A.L., Abbott, R., Hayhurst, H., Moore, R., and Garland, A.: Effects of cognitive therapy on psychological symptoms and social functioning in residual depression. *Br J Psychiat* 2000a; 177: 440–446.

Scott, J., Stanton, B., Garland, A., and Ferrier, I.N.: Cognitive vulnerability in patients with bipolar disorder. *Psychol Med* 2000b; 30: 467–72.

Scott, J., Paykel, E., Morriss, R., Bentall, R., Kinderman, P., Johnson, T., Abbott, R., and Haghurst, H.: Cognitive-behavioural therapy for same and recurrent bipolar disorders: randomised controlled trial. *Br J Psychiat* 2006; 188: 313–320.

Shakir, S.A., Volkmar, F.R., Bacon, S., and Pfefferbaum, A.: Group psychotherapy as an adjunct to lithium maintenance. *Am J Psychiat* 1979; 136: 455–456.

Spitz, H.I.: Principles of group and family therapy for depression and mania. In: Georgotas, A., Cancro, R. (eds.). *Depression and Mania*. New York: Elsevier, 1988.

Swartz, H.A., and Frank, E.: Psychotherapy for bipolar depression: a phase-specific treatment strategy? *Bipolar Disord* 2001; 3: 11–22.

Tohen, M., Tsuang, M.T., and Goodwin, D.C.: Prediction of outcome in mania by mood-congruent or mood-incongruent psychotic features. *Am J Psychiat* 1992; 149: 1580–1584.

Tsai, S.Y., Kuo, C.J., Chen, C.C., and Lee, H.C.: Risk factors for completed suicide in bipolar disorder. *J Clin Psychiat* 2002; 63: 469–476.

Van Gent, E.M.: Follow-up study of 3 years' group therapy with lithium treatment. *Encephale* 2000; 26: 76–79.

Van Gent, E.M., and Zwart, F.M.: Psychoeducation of partners of bipolar manic patients. *J Affect Disord* 1991; 21: 15–18.

Vieta, E., and Barcia, D.: El Trastorno Bipolar en el siglo XVIII [Bipolar disorder in the eighteenth century]. Madrid: MRA, 2000.

Vieta, E., and Cirera, E.: Trastornos bipolares organicos [Organic bipolar disorders]. In: Vieta, E., and Gastó, C. (eds.). *Trastornos Bipolares*. Barcelona: Springer-Verlag, 1997, pp. 479–495.

Vieta, E., Nieto, E., Gastó, C., and Cirera, E.: Serious suicide attempts in affective patients. *J Affect Disord* 1992; 24: 147–152.

Vieta, E., Gastó, C., Otero, A., Nieto, E., Menchón, J.M., and Vallejo, J.: Características clínicas del trasforno bipolar bipo II, una categoría válida de dificil diagnóstico. *Psiquiatría Biológica* 1994; 1: 104–110.

Vieta, E., Benabarre, A., Gastó, C., Nieto, E., Colom, F., Otero, A., and Vallejo, J.: Suicidal behavior in bipolar I and bipolar II disorder. *J Nerv Ment Dis* 1997a; 185: 407–409.

Vieta, E., Gastó, C., Martinez de Osaba, M.J., Nieto, E., Cantó, T.J., Otero, A., and Vallejo, J.: Prediction of depressive relapse in remitted bipolar patients using corticotrophin-releasing hormone challenge test. *Acta Psychiat Scand* 1997b; 95: 205–211.

Vieta, E., Gastó, C., Otero, A., Nieto, E., and Vallejo, J.: Differential features between bipolar I and bipolar II disorder. *Compr Psychiat* 1997c; 38: 98–101.

Vieta, E., Reinares, M., Corbella, B., Benabarre, A., Gilaberte, I., Colom, F., Martinez-Aran, A., Gasto, C., and Tohen, M.: Olanzapine as long-term adjunctive therapy in treatment-resistant bipolar disorder. *J Clin Psychopharmacol* 2001; 21: 469–473.

Volkmar, F.R., Bacon, S., Shakir, S.A., and Pfefferbaum, A.: Group therapy in the management of manic-depressive illness. *Am J Psychother* 1981; 35: 226–234.

Ward, E., King, M., Lloyd, M., Bower, P., Sibbald, B., Farrelly, S., Gabbay, M., Tarrier, N., and Addington-Hall, J.: Randomized controlled trial of nondirective counseling, cognitive–behavior therapy, and usual general practitioner care for patients with depression. I: clinical effectiveness. *Br Med J* 2000; 321: 1383–1388.

Wehr, T.A., Goodwin, F.K., Wirz-Justice, A., Breitmaier, J., and Craig, C.: Forty-eight-hour sleep-wake cycles in manic-depressive illness: naturalistic observations and sleep deprivation experiment. *Arch Gen Psychiat* 1982; 39: 559–565.

Wehr, T.A., Sack, D.A., and Rosenthal, N.E.: Sleep reduction as a final common pathway in the genesis of mania. *Am J Psychiat* 1987; 144: 210–214.

Weiss, R.D., Greenfield, S.F., Najavits, L.M., Soto, J.A., Wyner, D., Tohen, M. et al.: Medication adherence among patients with bipolar disorder and substance use disorder. *J Clin Psychiat* 1998; 59: 172–174.

Weiss, R., Griffin, M., and Greenfield, S.: Group therapy for patients with bipolar disorder and substance dependence: results of a pilot study. *J Clin Psychiat* 2000; 61: 361–367.

Winters, K., and Neale, J.: Mania and low self-esteem. *J Abnorm Psychol* 1985; 94: 282–290.

Woods, J.H., Katz, J.L., and Winger, G.: Use and abuse of benzodiazepines: issues relevant to prescribing. *J Am Med Assoc* 1988; 260: 3476–3480.

Wulsin, L., Bachop, M., and Hoffman, D.: Group therapy in manic-depressive illness. *Am J Psychother* 1988; 42: 263–271.

Wyatt, R.J., and Henter, I.: An economic evaluation of manic-depressive illness 1991. *Soc Psychiat Psychiat Epidemiol* 1995; 30: 213–219.

Yalom, I.D.: *The Theory and Practice of Group Psychotherapy*. New York: Basic Books, 1995.

## Recommended books

Goldberg, J.F., and Harrow, M. (eds.).: *Bipolar Disorders. Clinical Course and Outcome*. Washington, DC: American Psychiatric Press, 1999.

Lam, D.H., Jones, S.H., Hayward, P., and Bright, J.A.: *Cognitive Therapy for Bipolar Disorder*. Chichester: John Wiley & Sons Ltd., 1999.

# Index

Note: Page numbers in *italics* refer to figures and tables.